MW00792013

In this comprehensive review, the author challenging topic with wisdom and cl prompts for self-reflection that should be required reading for all therapists, as well as detailed practical advice for those doing forensic evaluations and expert testimony. A text for all mental health practitioners.

—**Judith L. Herman, MD,** Senior Lecturer in Psychiatry, Harvard Medical School, Cambridge, MA, United States

Dr. Pope and colleagues have produced a brave and searching work on an issue of critical importance to mental health professionals in every specialty area. It has long been a fantasy of my own that someone would write a book like this—one catering so directly to the needs of forensic practitioners as well as others. All readers will appreciate this book's wealth of appended practical resources.

—**Eric Y. Drogin, JD, PhD, ABPP (Forensic),** Affiliated Lead of Psycholegal Studies, Psychiatry, Law, and Society Program, Brigham and Women's Hospital, Harvard Medical School, Cambridge, MA, United States; Former President, American Board of Forensic Psychology; Former Chair, American Psychological Association Committee on Professional Practice and Standards

What a book! This brave and highly accessible work humanizes therapists' sexual feelings and fantasies in the context of culture, research, and the standard of care. Therapists and expert witnesses will find this meticulously researched book indispensable. I am delighted to have this groundbreaking resource for my clinical and forensic practice, supervision, and teaching.

—**Julie Goldenson, PhD,** Clinical and Forensic Psychologist; Assistant Professor, Department of Applied Psychology and Human Development, University of Toronto, Toronto, ON, Canada

Pope, Chavez-Dueñas, and Adames have done it again! These authors consistently set the bar for foundational texts that train psychologists and mental health providers. Their previous books on ethics and taboo topics in therapy are groundbreaking, helping us understand complex issues and develop ethically humane and socially just practices. Their latest volume, *Therapists' Sexual Feelings and Fantasies*, is a unique and indispensable resource that explores aspects often neglected in other works, such as power dynamics, gender, race, and sexual orientation. The authors masterfully contextualize the ethical and legal issues surrounding therapist–client sexual interactions. I appreciate the accessible language, real-life examples, and helpful resources typical of their work. This book is simply terrific. It is a foundational and innovative text that sets a new standard in the field and is a must-read for practitioners of any theoretical orientation.

—**Helen A. Neville, PhD,** Professor, Educational Psychology and African American Studies, University of Illinois Urbana-Champaign, Champaign, IL, United States; 2023–2024 President, Society of Counseling Psychology

Therapists' Sexual Feelings and Fantasies addresses the challenging topic of therapists' sexual feelings about people with whom they work. It offers a much-needed, contemporary, expansive perspective. It provides a positive, normalizing, and realistic consideration of sexual feelings, including vulnerabilities. This extraordinary contribution gives readers a remarkable set of resources and tools to help deal with clinical and forensic work in this area. The authors, who are ethicists, provide rich, thought-provoking questions. This book is a superb treasure beneficial for all practitioners. I give it my highest recommendation.

—**Melba J. T. Vasquez, PhD, ABPP,** independent practice, Austin, TX, United States; Former President, American Psychological Association

This book goes beyond what we all learn about boundary violations, emphasizing the personal skill and professional competence that is required to embrace and manage our natural but conflictual sexual feelings in relating to our patients. The authors promote systematic personal reflection throughout the book and delineate potential vulnerabilities to problematic relationships. The one book every therapist should read.

—**Jon G. Allen, PhD,** Clinical Professor, Voluntary Faculty, Menninger Department of Psychiatry and Behavioral Sciences, Baylor College of Medicine, Houston, TX, United States

In this courageous book, the authors provide nuanced and informed discussion and resources to help therapists and forensic evaluators wade through the maelstrom of romantic and sexual feelings. They discuss the deplorable intellectual history of therapist–patient sexual involvement, and the ongoing vulnerabilities of contemporary therapists. They provide honest acknowledgment of intense therapist reactions, while describing steps to avoid the sexual and/or emotional abuse of patients. They also cover forensic issues in cases of suspected therapist–patient sex and provide evolving resources for informed consent, the review of treatment plans, and other practical matters that will help make psychotherapy a healthier arena for therapists and patients alike.

—**Etzel Cardeña, PhD,** Thorsen Professor in Psychology, Lund University, Lund, Sweden

This book addresses one of the key neglected issues in practicing ethically and effectively. The authors' combination of experience, a willingness to approach very sensitive topics, and practical guidelines should be required reading for all psychotherapists in training. In fact, there are few psychotherapists, however long they have practiced and whatever their theoretical persuasion, who will not benefit from studying the advice and resources this book contains.

—**Chris R. Brewin, PhD,** Emeritus Professor of Clinical Psychology, University College London, London, United Kingdom

Therapists' Sexual Feelings and Fantasies

Therapists' Sexual Feelings and Fantasies

Research, Practice,
Ethics, and Forensics

Kenneth S. Pope
Nayeli Y. Chavez-Dueñas
Hector Y. Adames

 AMERICAN PSYCHOLOGICAL ASSOCIATION

The opinions and statements published are the responsibility of the authors, and such opinions and statements do not necessarily represent the policies of the American Psychological Association.

Published by
American Psychological Association
750 First Street, NE
Washington, DC 20002
https://www.apa.org

Order Department
https://www.apa.org/pubs/books
order@apa.org

Typeset in Charter and Interstate by Circle Graphics, Inc., Reisterstown, MD

Printer: Gasch Printing, Odenton, MD
Cover Designer: Gwen J. Grafft, Minneapolis, MN
Cover Concept: Hector Y. Adames, Chicago, IL

Library of Congress Cataloging-in-Publication Data

Names: Pope, Kenneth S., author. | Chavez-Dueñas, Nayeli Y., author. |
  Adames, Hector Y., author. | American Psychological Association, issuing body.
Title: Therapists' sexual feelings and fantasies : research, practice,
  ethics, and forensics / by Kenneth S. Pope, Nayeli Y. Chavez-Dueñas,
  Hector Y. Adames.
Description: Washington, DC : American Psychological Association, [2025] |
  Includes bibliographical references and index.
Identifiers: LCCN 2024029810 (print) | LCCN 2024029811 (ebook) |
  ISBN 9781433844331 (paperback) | ISBN 9781433844348 (ebook)
Subjects: MESH: Professional-Patient Relations | Sexual Behavior--ethics |
  Ethics, Professional | Countertransference | Forensic Psychiatry--methods
Classification: LCC RC343 (print) | LCC RC343 (ebook) | NLM WM 62 |
  DDC 174/.961689--dc23/eng/20241010
LC record available at https://lccn.loc.gov/2024029810
LC ebook record available at https://lccn.loc.gov/2024029811

https://doi.org/10.1037/0000443-000

Printed in the United States of America

10 9 8 7 6 5 4 3 2 1

We dedicate this book to the victims and survivors of sexual violations in psychotherapy relationships. May you find peace in knowing it was never your fault and hold on to the hope of rebuilding meaningful and trustworthy connections.

Contents

Acknowledgments

We are deeply indebted to and profoundly thankful for the many special people and communities—professors, supervisors, mentors, colleagues, patients, students, friends, family, professional and social groups and organizations—who have meant so much to us on our life journey and professional paths. You have inspired us with your kindness, thoughtfulness, courage, and support. You have lifted us when our spirits were dragging along the ground, challenged us when our sights were too low and we were giving less than our best effort, and showed us the difference that a life well lived can mean for the individual and for so many others.

We also want to thank those whose invaluable contributions—ideas, research, critiques, articles, and volumes—we cite in this book. It's a cliché, but in this case, it's apt: We stand on the shoulders of giants.

We express our sincere appreciation to Phil Brakefield; Ronald V. Hall, MD; Maryam M. Jernigan, PhD; Karen Olio, MA; Katherine Pope, PhD; Shweta Sharma, PsyD; and Swati Sharma, who provided feedback and helped us pick the book cover that captures the essence of our work and makes us smile at how beautiful it is.

We would never have been able to create this book without the skilled guidance and support of Susan Reynolds at American Psychological Association (APA) Books. We also thank Molly Gage, Rohita Atluri, Erin O'Brien, Lina Rainone, and everyone at APA Books who helped bring this project together. Your expertise was just the alchemy that our manuscript needed.

Therapists' Sexual Feelings and Fantasies

INTRODUCTION

The Elephant in the Therapy Office

The psychotherapy profession has struggled to deal openly, honestly, and effectively with therapists' sexual feelings, fantasies, and behaviors. We wrote this book to provide a brief, practical guide for therapists and expert witnesses to the complex, difficult issues in this area, focusing on three different aspects:

- therapists' experiences of sexual attraction and related phenomena (e.g., fantasies, dreams, arousal) toward their clients,
- therapists' violations of sexual boundaries with their clients (e.g., therapist–patient sexual involvement), and
- therapists testifying in cases where therapist–patient sex is at issue.

The book reviews the research and current knowledge but also draws this information together to help therapists and both fact and expert witnesses do their work more effectively.

The topics are challenging. The book examines how the normal, natural experience of sexual attraction to a client often, according to the research, evokes feelings of anxiety, guilt, and confusion in the therapist who has done nothing wrong. It reviews the field's early history—in some ways not so long

https://doi.org/10.1037/0000443-001
Therapists' Sexual Feelings and Fantasies: Research, Practice, Ethics, and Forensics,
by K. S. Pope, N. Y. Chavez-Dueñas, and H. Y. Adames

3

ago—of enforcing intentional blindness to therapists' sexual involvement with clients, suppressing research findings, and attempting to expel those who would publish findings. It documents how a wide variety of famous therapists—many still quoted as authorities—started sexual relationships with their clients.

The book's three authors come from diverse backgrounds, have different perspectives, and work from different theoretical orientations. We believe that bringing together these backgrounds and weaving in our perspectives and orientations enriches what the book has to offer.

A note on terminology: For brevity, we use the terms therapist, psycho-therapist, and counselor interchangeably rather than listing or hyphenating all three. Some therapists think of the people they serve as "clients," while others use the term "patients." Again, for the sake of brevity, we use these terms interchangeably.

PART I

A POSITIVE APPROACH TO THERAPISTS' SEXUAL FEELINGS AND FANTASIES

1 A POSITIVE, OPEN, AND HONEST APPROACH TO THERAPISTS' SEXUAL FEELINGS

Sexual feelings are inescapable for many of us. They are one of the most natural and shared human experiences, yet they are often challenging and awkward to discuss. In psychotherapy, as in life, sexual feelings are sometimes unavoidable, and when they surface, we might be at a loss for how to navigate this experience competently, confidently, ethically, and helpfully.

If sexual feelings are common, why are they challenging to talk about openly? Why do they often stir up confusion, anxiety, guilt, denial, and distortions?

The answers to these questions can be vast, including the possibility that, given the history of our field, therapists worry their sexual feelings may lead to unethical and harmful behaviors and outcomes. Or they may fear that colleagues may see them as unprofessional. Or these feelings may be associated with therapists who have made wild and empty claims that they can heal through sexual acts with their patients. Or, or, or. . . .

To echo our opening statement, having sexual feelings in psychotherapy is common. Handled correctly, they can inform and enrich our work with clients. Mishandled, they may lead us to violate ethical, legal, clinical, and

https://doi.org/10.1037/0000443-002
Therapists' Sexual Feelings and Fantasies: Research, Practice, Ethics, and Forensics,
by K. S. Pope, N. Y. Chavez-Dueñas, and H. Y. Adames

professional responsibilities and place our clients at risk for significant harm (see Chapter 5). These responsibilities hold not only for us as individuals but also on the institutional level. Consider how professional organizations have sometimes covered up the data and protected offenders, as described and documented in later chapters.

WHERE ARE WE GOING WITH ALL THIS AND WHY?

This book is a practical, research-based guide to understanding the reactions sketched in the opening paragraph and approaching sexual feelings and fantasies in psychotherapy with more openness, directness, and honesty. Several excellent articles and books have provided information focusing on (a) therapists' sexual feelings, (b) therapist–patient sexual involvement, or (c) preparing forensic reports or testifying as an expert or fact witness in legal cases relevant to this area. However, the interplay among these three areas is often not considered, and each domain tends to be discussed outside the crucial context of the other area.

In this book, we aim to build on the existing knowledge and provide essential information and guidance in all three areas so that each may be understood in fuller context and in relation to the other.

A Positive Approach to Sexual Feelings

We organized the book into seven sections. The first section encourages a positive approach that views our sexual feelings as a valuable resource that informs and enriches our understanding, competence, and effectiveness as therapists. When we are aware and accepting of our sexual or romantic attraction to, arousal in the presence of, or erotic fantasies about a client, it helps us understand what is going on in our experience as therapists and in our relationship with the client. In the first section, we

- summarize what history teaches us about therapists' sexual feelings and our reactions to them;
- describe barriers to good practice;
- discuss therapists' sexual fantasies;
- explore critical sociohistorical contexts essential to understanding therapists' sexual feelings; and
- examine the influence of power dynamics, gender, sexual orientation, and race.

Therapist-Patient Sexual Involvement

The book's second section focuses on therapist–patient sexual involvement. The chapters in this section offer concise discussions of the following topics:

- evolving ethical and legal standards,
- the influence of Zoom and other digital platforms on therapist–patient sexual involvement,
- red flags that we may be edging toward sexual involvement with a patient,
- common ways therapists try to justify to themselves and others their sexual involvement with patients,
- key issues to keep in mind if a patient tells us they were sexually involved with a prior therapist, and
- a comprehensive approach to preventing therapist–patient sexual involvement.

Forensic Work Involving Therapists' Sexual Behaviors With Clients

The third section focuses on forensics. It addresses important points for therapists to know and consider so they do not enter the courtroom's adversarial arena unprepared. In this brief guide to the unique rules, risks, and challenges of consulting, preparing forensic reports, or testifying in civil, criminal, or administrative legal cases involving therapists' sexual behaviors with clients, we tackle the following areas:

- identifying cognitive and emotional biases and other reactions in therapists–patient sex forensic work,
- working with attorneys,
- testifying as a fact witness about a client or former client, and
- testifying as an expert witness.

Resources to Meet the Challenges of Clinical and Forensic Work

The final four sections of the book offer tools designed to address the complexities encountered in clinical and forensic work when therapist–patient sexual involvement occurs, including:

- informed consent resources;
- tools for reviewing treatment plans and notes; and
- tools for preparing for deposition, cross-examination, subpoenas, and compelled testimony.

OVERCOMING DISCONNECTS–AN INVITATION

Acknowledging sexual feelings or romantic attractions toward a client is not easy. You may get to the end of the book and not see yourself in it. Perhaps you'll feel the content is essential but does not capture your experiences. While this book provides valuable information on sexual feelings and romantic attractions toward clients, acquiring knowledge on the topic is only the initial part of the journey to connect with the material honestly.

In many ways, some past and continuing problems in this area result from our disconnection with the material. We may have completed the monumental task of reading all the history, theory, and research on this topic and understand all the relevant legislation, case law, ethical standards, licensing regulations, and professional guidelines but still experience difficulties, make avoidable mistakes, and fail to help our clients because we've not engaged fully with the information. We might have gained an impressive, intellectualized understanding of this area, but the topic remains abstract and isolated, cut off from our immediate personal experience.

It is as if we had read every book on grief and loss we could lay our hands on. We read great writing on the experience of grief and loss, reviewed examples of their various forms, and understood their stages. However, when we think about these experiences, we often think about others navigating grief and loss. We can come up with many examples of how these experiences have impacted people around us. Still, pausing, facing, and imagining ourselves experiencing profound grief and loss is hard. We may avoid thinking about these topics, and if something happens that reminds us of our losses, we may try to think about something else out of fear of what would happen if we honestly acknowledged how loss impacts our lives. In these moments, we resort to disconnecting from the loss.

This book offers an invitation for you to connect to a topic that many of us are socialized to avoid thinking about, naming, and discussing, but that is a common part of the human experience: sexual feelings and romantic attractions in psychotherapy. This book goes beyond simply providing facts and knowledge; it aims to support you on this journey to overcoming the disconnect. It offers guidance and the opportunity to engage with the material personally and meaningfully. To this end, each chapter closes with scenarios and questions that may help you self-reflect on the various topics discussed.

Let's begin the journey.

- How might your unique constellation of identities (e.g., cultural, sexual, spiritual, political), personal history, attitudes, beliefs, values, preferences, and biases affect how you engage with the material in this book on a personal level?

- Are there ways these identities make full engagement and immediacy easier or harder?

- Do you have any characteristic ways of avoiding engagement? If so, how could you work with them to lessen the avoidance?

Consider your graduate program and internship.

- How much information did you receive on the theory and research on therapists' sexual feelings (including sexual attraction to a client, sexual arousal during a therapy session, and sexual fantasies about a client), and how can these feelings be a valuable resource when approached positively and knowledgeably?

- How much coverage did you receive on the theory, research, ethics, law, and professional standards regarding therapist–patient sexual involvement?

- How much supervised experience did you receive in this area?

- How much coverage did you receive about conducting a clinical assessment of a patient who alleges sexual behavior with a prior therapist?

- How much coverage did you receive about conducting a forensic psychological assessment of a patient who alleges sexual behavior with a prior therapist?

- How much coverage did you receive about testifying as a fact witness regarding your client if they alleged sexual activity with another therapist or testifying as an expert witness about someone who was not your client but who alleges sexual contact with a therapist?

- To what degree do you consider yourself knowledgeable, competent, and well-prepared to practice in these three areas?

Imagine you are sitting in the cafeteria of a large hospital and mental health center when two men sit down at a nearby table for coffee. It becomes clear that both are therapists. At one point, you hear one say to the other, "Man, you should've seen the client who showed up for therapy this morning. She was hot. And the way she was dressed! Full-time seduction. I'd never mess with a client, but I gotta confess, I see why some therapists might think it would be worth the risk."

- What feelings do you experience as you imagine this scenario?

- What thoughts do you have?

- Are you tempted to turn around to see what these guys look like, if only so that you can recognize them if your professional paths ever cross?

- What do you imagine these guys look like—age, race or ethnicity, clothing?

- Did you form any mental image of the client in this scenario? If so, what did you see? What was the client's approximate age, income, education level, clothing style, race, or ethnicity?

- According to the information and your experience, what is the probability that you would react similarly to seeing the client dressed in a "seductive" or "sexy" manner? What are the probabilities that she'd be dressed in a conservative business suit appropriate to chairing a board meeting of a Fortune 500 company or addressing a religious congregation? What are the chances that she is dressed in baggy sweatpants and a long-sleeved baggy sweatshirt and hoodie?

- When a client is described in rounds, a chart note, or a forensic report as flirty, sexually teasing, forward, provocative, coy, seductive, kittenish, or alluring, what are your thoughts? What are your feelings?

Imagine your first patient at the university mental health clinic is an undocumented graduate student who, as you discuss what prompted them to reach out for help, discloses that they were sexually abused when they were 8 years old by another therapist in your area. This alleged therapist is a highly respected colleague who continues practicing, teaching, and supervising. They also tell you that if you tell anyone, it will likely lead to outing them as undocumented, terminating their graduate studies, and likely lead to deportation.

- What do you feel as you imagine yourself in this scenario?

- What are your thoughts?

- What possible courses of action do you consider, and what are the likely outcomes and pros and cons of each?

- Which do you think you would choose and why?

- What is the first thing you would say to this client?

- Are you aware of the legislation, case law, ethical standards, and professional or licensing requirements for mandatory child abuse reporting in your area?

- How would you chart this or discuss it in rounds or with a supervisor?

- If you disclosed it in rounds or supervision to any other clinician and had not already filed a formal report, would they be legally required to report it?

- If you disclosed it in written form in your chart note and had not filed a formal report and another clinician read it, would they be legally required to report it?

- Would your responses to the previous items change if you found out that the patient is a widowed parent with no other living relatives and who, if deported, would likely be separated from the two children they are raising?

Imagine you are asked to conduct a forensic assessment of an adult suing their psychotherapist, alleging therapist–patient sexual involvement.

- How many hours would you estimate the assessment might take? If it's hard to narrow down, what's the least and the most amount of time you might need to allot for a good forensic assessment?

- Would you include any standardized assessment instruments in your evaluation? If so, which ones?

- Do you assess whether the person is dissembling, exaggerating, or trying to mislead in any way? If so, how?

- If you were asked to determine how the person was harmed, the extent of the harm, the cost of the damages, and the anticipated cost of future treatment for the harm caused by the therapist–patient sex, which of those would you attempt to answer and how?

- Would you anticipate any particularly challenging cross-examination questions? If so, what steps, would you take to prepare to respond to those questions?

- Suppose a fellow therapist asked you to conduct a clinical assessment (rather than a forensic assessment) as part of a treatment planning process. In that case, unrelated to any legal action, would your approach or methods differ in any way?

Imagine that you are asked to conduct a forensic assessment of a psychotherapist who has been accused of becoming sexually involved with a patient and is facing both a malpractice suit and criminal charges.

- How many hours would you estimate the assessment might take? If it's hard to narrow down, what's the least and most amount of time you might need to allot for a good forensic assessment?

- Would you include any standardized assessment instruments in your evaluation? If so, which ones?

- Would you attempt to assess whether the person is dissembling, exaggerating, or trying to mislead in any way? If so, how?

- Would you anticipate any particularly challenging cross-examination questions? If so, what steps, if any, would you take to prepare to respond to those questions?

- Suppose a fellow therapist asked you to conduct a clinical assessment (rather than a forensic assessment) as part of a treatment planning process. In that case, unrelated to any legal action, would your approach or methods differ in any way?

A common theme we'll keep coming back to throughout the book is that having sexual and romantic feelings toward clients is an experience shared among most, if not all, therapists at one time or another. Recognizing that these experiences are natural and human can free us from the stigma and guilt associated with them. It enables us to focus on the work that matters and discover or create ways to develop a positive approach to handling sexual and romantic feelings in our work as therapists.

2 INFLUENTIAL THERAPISTS WHO HAVE ENGAGED IN SEX WITH CLIENTS AND WHY IT MATTERS

The Importance of Sociohistorical Context

Understanding most topics requires a thorough grasp of the context in which they take place. In this chapter, we discuss influential therapists who have engaged in sex with clients and why it matters. We begin by hearing directly from nationally known psychologist Gerry Koocher, who stated:

> On occasion, I tell my students and professional audiences that I once spent an entire psychotherapy session holding hands with a 26-year-old woman together in a quiet darkened room. That disclosure usually elicits more than a few gasps and grimaces. When I add that I could not bring myself to end the session after 50 minutes and stayed with the young woman holding hands for another half hour, and when I add the fact that I never billed for the extra time, eyes roll. (2006, p. xxii)

Although Chapter 3 focuses on fantasies, it's worth pausing here to ask readers about your fantasies as you begin reading this chapter. What is your fantasy about what is going on? Why is Gerry behaving in this way with this woman? Where do you think this is headed? Could you imagine yourself ever doing something like this during a clinical session?

https://doi.org/10.1037/0000443-003
Therapists' Sexual Feelings and Fantasies: Research, Practice, Ethics, and Forensics, by K. S. Pope, N. Y. Chavez-Dueñas, and H. Y. Adames

It is difficult—perhaps impossible—to understand what is going on free of the context. Gerry adds some essential background:

> Then I explain that the young woman had cystic fibrosis with severe pulmonary disease and panic-inducing air hunger. She had to struggle through three breaths on an oxygen line before she could speak a sentence. I had come into her room, sat down by her bedside, and asked how I might help her. She grabbed my hand and said, "Don't let go." When the time came for another appointment, I called a nurse to take my place. (Koocher, 2006, p. xxii)

This narrative illustrates a central theme of this book: When considering a therapist's fantasies or behavior, context is key. It is so easy for us to wrongly assume that we are adequately aware of the context, leading us to misunderstand and misjudge the situation. The late psychologist Daniel Kahneman, recipient of the Nobel Prize, described this kind of mistake as the unfounded belief in WYSIATI: What you see is all there is (Kahneman, 2011, p. 85). It is always worth asking what important information could be missing and how to find it. If it is unavailable, how can you at least consider what is missing? If we fail to ask this question and simply assume that what we see or know is all there is or at least all that's important, all too often, we are off to the races, headed in the wrong direction, with all sorts of fallacies and biases (e.g., conformation bias) strengthening our misinformation and misjudgments and protecting us from any disconfirming facts, theories, or other ways of understanding what is going on.

Though this theme of critically attending to adequate and accurate context runs throughout the book, Chapter 4 will pay special attention to contexts such as power, gender, sexual orientation, and race. In this chapter, we focus closely on the sociohistorical context. Two aspects of this context seem particularly relevant:

- How little research has been published focusing on therapists' sexual fantasies about their clients, leaving the field lacking a firm and extensive empirical base to help understand this phenomenon and its implications.

- How, despite a prohibition against therapist–patient sex that predates the Hippocratic Oath, some of the most famous and influential therapists have engaged in sex with their patients, presenting us with a tangle of difficult questions, including how their sexual involvement with patients influenced the field and how we understand and discuss therapist–patient sexual involvement.

The following section provides some background information for the first aspect mentioned earlier regarding therapists' sexual fantasies about their clients.

A FREUDIAN START, A WATSONIAN STOP

We can gain a better understanding of therapists' sexual fantasies by viewing the topic from a sociohistorical perspective. Freud came close to pioneering the discussion of therapists' sexual fantasies when, in the course of describing clients' transference in the form of falling in love with the therapist, he emphasized the importance of the therapist keeping their countertransference in check (Freud, 1912/1915; see also Freud, 1910/1924). Around the same time, John B. Watson (1913, 1914, 1919, 1925) was leading a major shift in American psychology away from studying fantasies, consciousness, and inner experience. Instead, he advocated theory and research that focused on external, observable behavior. Roger Brown (1958) described this phase of psychology and stated, "In 1913 John Watson mercifully closed the bloodshot inner eye of American psychology. With great relief the profession trained its exteroceptors on the laboratory animal" (p. 93). Even the lasting influence of Freudian thought and psychoanalysis, which prioritized the inner life of individuals, did not lead to substantial research into the sexual fantasies of therapists. This might be attributed, in part, to Freudian's emphasis on the unconscious mind and a hydraulic-like system of drives or other forces of which individuals were often unaware. It was not until the 1960s and 1970s that the focus began to shift to research on consciousness (Holt, 1964; Neisser, 1967; Paivio, 1971; Pope & Singer, 1978; Segal, 1971; Sheehan, 1972; Singer, 1975a, 1975b), laying the groundwork for scientific approaches to studying sexual fantasies. However, critics continued to discount this trend as a "diverting preoccupation with a supposed or real inner life" (Skinner, 1975, p. 46).

Influential Therapists Who Engaged in Sex With Their Clients

Therapist–patient sexual involvement has been a concern since the beginning of the "talking cure." The history of the field includes numerous instances of therapists engaging in sexual behaviors with their clients. In this chapter, we summarize some documented cases of prominent, influential, and still frequently cited therapists who engaged in sexual activities with their patients.

Let's begin with Sándor Ferenczi, a close friend and frequent traveling companion of Sigmund Freud. Ferenczi was a member of the Vienna Psychoanalytic Society, the world's oldest psychoanalytic society, and president of the International Psychoanalytical Association (Brabant et al., 1993; Falzeder et al., 1996, 2000). In 1909, Ferenczi wrote to Freud describing that he'd become sexually involved with a patient. He confessed he was ambivalent about the whole thing because, as Ferenczi had told the patient, she seemed too old for him, and he still found himself sexually attracted to younger women (Pope, 1994). He later began treating the woman's daughter as his patient, fell in love with the daughter, and told the mother and daughter that he would be marrying the daughter.

Ferenczi became ambivalent once again and could not decide whether he wanted to marry the patient who was the mother or the patient who was the daughter. Ferenczi concluded that what he had learned from serving as the daughter's therapist convinced him that she was not the sort of woman who was stable enough (!) for marriage. Nevertheless, he still enjoyed sex with her. However, while Ferenczi enjoyed spending time with the mother, he did not find her to be an attractive, exciting, or satisfying sexual partner, in his not-at-all-humble opinion. Ferenczi wrote that he tried living with both women in a threesome as an experiment, but it did not work out. He decided to satisfy his sexual urges by purchasing the services of sex workers (Pope, 1994).

Ferenczi continued to exchange letters with Freud, seeking guidance with this dilemma. He complained, with no hint of irony or self-reflection, that his psychoanalysis of the daughter seemed to have gotten bogged down and was moving slowly.

Before continuing the chapter, it is worth noticing Freud's main reactions and conclusions. As you read this material, note how you react. Does Freud's response surprise you in any way? To what degree do you believe some contemporary therapists might respond in the same way in a similar situation? How do you think you would react in this situation?

When the mother consulted him, Freud impressed on her that she must at all costs not tell anyone else about her psychoanalysis or the situation with Ferenczi. After seeing the daughter in treatment, Freud reached three major conclusions that seem, unfortunately, all too often to echo throughout the history of the field, down to and including the present, when patients who have been sexually involved with a therapist seek subsequent therapy or consultation.

- Freud interpreted the daughter's desire for revenge as resistance to the therapy.

- Freud described the key element of the daughter's character as manifest narcissism.

- Freud found the daughter's central or presenting problem to be quite simple and obvious, concluding that she suffered from a neurotic compulsion to fall in love with doctors (Pope, 1994).

How would you describe the main themes that emerged from this description? Do you see these themes arising in contemporary situations involving abuse of power or sexual exploitation?

Ernest Jones, a colleague of Freud and Ferenczi, is another famous thera-pist who engaged in sexual activity with a patient. Jones was Freud's first English-speaking follower and a member of Freud's inner circle. Jones founded the *International Journal of Psychoanalysis*, served two terms as president of the International Psychoanalytical Association, and founded the London Psycho-analytical Society (later the British Psychoanalytical Society) and the American Psychoanalytic Association. Jones faced a threat from one of his patients, who threatened to make public her account of sexual involvement with him during his time as her analyst. When Jones found out about his client's intent, he arranged to pay her $500 as part of a "gag agreement" in which she would agree to keep quiet, not mention what happened to her to anyone, and avoid involving him in a scandal (Hale, 1971).

Carl Jung served as the first president of the International Psychoanalytical Association and was initially seen as a key figure who could advance the field following Sigmund Freud's departure. However, Jung grew discontent with psychoanalysis and founded his own school of analytical psychology. Histor-ical records indicate that Jung had complex relationships with some of his patients, including sexual involvement with several of his patients. One case involved a patient who sought advice from Freud about her interactions with Jung. In response, Jung falsely reassured both Freud and the patient's mother that no sexual misconduct had occurred. Freud's response to the woman encompasses three central themes, which include

- that Jung was incapable of such unethical behavior and so was innocent of her accusations;

- that it would be best for her to blot out all memories and thoughts related to this matter and try never to think of it again; and

- that this matter must remain secret, and she should never discuss it with anyone else (Pope, 1994).

Unfortunately, Ferenczi, Jones, and Jung are only a small sample of the prominent therapists who crossed the line. Other famous therapists who have engaged in sexual behaviors with patients include the following:

- Otto Fenichel
- Horace Frink
- Frieda Fromm-Reichman
- Georg Groddeck
- Otto Gross
- Karen Horney
- Fritz Perls

- Wilhelm Reich
- Ernst Simmel
- Wilhelm Stekel
- Harry Stack Sullivan
- Victor Tausk (Blechner, 2021; Hornstein, 2000; Levin, 2021; Shepherd, 1975; Strean, 2018; Warner, 1994)

A Therapist's Fame and Influence Does Not Justify Sexually Exploiting Clients

It has been hard for the field to come to grips with the fact that famous, influential, often-cited, well-respected therapists have violated their clients' trust and engaged in sexual activities with them. Unfortunately, the literature is sparse on how the sexual behavior of these therapists is best understood, how it affects our understanding of their teachings, and how it has influenced the evolution of the field.

The difficulty accepting this reality has contributed to this issue being ignored or disappearing into the profession's memory hole as if it never existed. Blechner (2021) examined reactions to prominent therapists engaging in sex with their patients and found that a disturbing theme tended to run through them. Reactions seemed to embody the belief that the safest and best course of action (for the therapist and the profession, not for the patient) was to keep quiet and not discuss it. Similarly, in a chapter titled "Don't Tell Anyone," Slochower (2021) wrote:

> Nearly all of us have been privy to gossip—and fact—about boundary violations (sexual and nonsexual). Yet only a tiny number of these violations have come under public scrutiny; even when they do, they are almost never openly discussed, let alone made public in wider forums. (pp. 143–144)

Silence in the profession about therapists' behaviors that have harmed their clients, such as sexual behaviors with clients, needs to be disrupted. Silence enables perpetrators, betrays victims, and undermines professional integrity. These issues, like all clinical, ethical, legal, and professional issues, should always be open to discussion and reconsideration.

Moreover, it is important to remember that "it was a famous person who did it" never justifies a violation of ethics and our responsibility to do no harm. That Freud used cocaine with his patients does not justify using it with our patients. When a prominent psychologist, whose attention-grabbing research appeared in *Science* and other prestigious journals over 3 decades and was covered in newspapers around the world and who held influential positions at three universities, was found to have "falsified data and made up entire experiments" (Carey, 2011, para. 1), it in no way offers justification for the rest us to lie and cheat in similar ways. Another prominent psychologist served as dean and was known as a rainmaker for bringing in huge grants. However, the cheering from universities at his seemingly miraculous work died down when his license was suspended. A plea agreement was reached on charges including mail fraud, tax evasion, conspiracy to commit money laundering, and conspiracy to impede and impair the Internal Revenue Service. He was sentenced to over 5 years in prison (Rodriguez, 2014). His fame and influence offer no justification for his behavior.

It is also important to acknowledge, when considering therapists who married their patients, that marriage is not, per se, justification for the rightness or acceptability of what goes on in the marriage. To use the most obvious examples, a person may deceive, dominate, belittle, humiliate, gaslight, batter, or rape a spouse, and the fact that the two people are married in no way justifies the behavior.

What Can We Do?

How can we begin to come to terms with a field in which some of the most famous, influential, often-cited, and admired therapists have violated a fundamental clinical, ethical, legal, and professional responsibility? Perhaps to remind ourselves that we are part of a human profession, and all of us have human weaknesses. Those who have engaged in sex with a patient are not part of some other group completely separate from and unlike us. We are all flawed human beings. Moreover, having exceptional talent, creativity, genius, accomplishments, fame, influence, and a substantial fan following cannot and will not provide immunity against making choices that compromise clinical, ethical, and professional values, potentially endangering a patient in the process and causing harm.

Second, we can become aware of how learning that a trusted and admired authority in the discipline has betrayed their clients' trust and the profession's ethics affects us as fellow therapists or just as fellow humans. What are our feelings, if any, when we learn that someone we and others looked up to engaged in sex with a patient? How, if at all, does it affect our trust?

Third, we can reflect on our patterns of strengths and weaknesses, strategies of denial, areas of temptation and rationalization, and tendencies to drift or lurch into bad decisions to do something wrong. If we can be open about these patterns, strategies, areas, and tendencies with ourselves and then perhaps with others, we may be better prepared to meet the pressures, temptations, and other challenges of our work. We can also work to grow and exercise our strengths, shore up our weaknesses, and improve our decision making.

Fourth, we can set aside the seemingly safe, traditional "vow of silence" and start speaking more directly, honestly, and courageously on these critical topics (see Pope et al., 2023). A clear and well-defined path forward is articulated by Blechner (2021), who emphasizes that

> We need to relax the unspoken but powerful ban on discussing this issue, in current clinical work and in the history [of our field]. Our message must shift: Don't keep quiet; speak out! We must resolve the dissociation between what we say publicly and think privately and what we believe unconsciously. Only when we deal with this gap can we hope to confront sexual boundary violations honestly and effectively. (p. 168)

Awakenings

The injunction to speak has not, so far, been heeded. In fact, the profession's conspiracy of silence about therapist–patient sexual involvement has been alive and at work for decades. You might be curious about what prompted a more conscious effort to discuss this phenomenon or what shook the profession awake into acknowledging the reality of therapist–patient sexual involvement. The answer to this question is sad and disappointing but predictable. It took patients filing lawsuits against their therapists alleging patient–therapist sexual involvement (e.g., *Roy v. Hartogs*, 1976; *Zipkin v. Freeman*, 1968). These lawsuits caught the attention of therapists and the public. Some had real financial consequences. For example, Evelyn Walker sued a prominent La Jolla psychiatrist, Zane Parzen, resulting in a $4,631,666 award for the plaintiff (Walker & Young, 1986). Evelyn Walker vividly described her experiences in *A Killing Cure* (Walker & Young, 1986).

Books, often written or coauthored by women who'd sued their therapists, provided vivid individual accounts. These books often quoted from chart notes, depositions, and trial testimony. Trailblazing books that contributed significantly to raising awareness about this topic include the following, listed in chronological order:

- *Betrayal: The True Story of the First Woman to Successfully Sue Her Psychiatrist for Using Sex in the Guise of Therapy* (Freeman & Roy, 1976)
- *Therapist* (Plasil, 1985)
- *A Killing Cure* (Walker & Young, 1986)
- *Sex in the Therapy Hour: A Case of Professional Incest* (Bates & Brodsky, 1989)
- *Abus de Pouvoir* [*Abuse of Power*] (Frennette, 1991)
- *You Must Be Dreaming* (Noël & Watterson, 1992)

These books played a part in waking up the field to the reality of therapist–patient sex and the harm that can result, but *You Must Be Dreaming* hit particularly hard because the therapist was internationally known psychiatrist and psychoanalyst Jules H. Masserman. Masserman had served as president of

- the American Psychiatric Association,
- the American Society for Group Psychotherapy,
- the American Association for Social Psychiatry,
- the Society of Biological Psychiatry, and
- the American Academy of Psychoanalysis.

He had chaired the Department of Psychiatry at Northwestern University and had written a dozen books, published over 400 articles, and received many honors (Pace, 1994).

Singer and composer Barbara Noël wrote a book and later a made-for-TV movie about her experiences as Masserman's patient, which included waking up suddenly during an IV sodium amytal session on the therapist's couch to find Masserman was raping her while she had been unconscious (Noël & Watterson, 1992).

Maintaining his innocence, Masserman settled four similar malpractice suits filed by his female patients. When Barbara Noël filed a formal complaint with the Illinois Psychiatric Society, it investigated and ruled against Masserman, suspending him. He appealed his case to the American Psychiatric Association but was unsuccessful.

Lawsuits and books about therapist–patient involvement caught the attention of the profession and the public, making both aware of the topic. Television movies were made based on the *Roy v. Hartogs* case and the book *You Must Be Dreaming*, and popular actors, including Sir Alec Guinness, Meryl Streep, John Huston, Christine Baransky, Roy Scheider, Dudley Moore, and David Strathairn, appeared in movies in which therapist–patient sex was central to the plot (e.g., *Lovesick, Still of the Night*). The topic was reflected in the highly rated television show *60 Minutes* (Rather, 1978) and the popular newspaper advice column Dear Abby (Van Buren, 1978).

The historical narrative presented in this chapter is undeniably challenging, but it's a challenge we must confront. By exposing, revisiting, and breaking the stubborn silence around therapist–patient sexual involvement, we can begin to understand and develop strategies to protect the public by preventing these boundary violations. Our professional responsibility is to provide the highest quality care to the people we serve. This includes our responsibility as practitioners to be fully aware of our discipline's history— both its successes and failures—to minimize the risk of repeating past mistakes like the ones committed by the influential therapists we discussed in the chapter.

An Invitation for Self-Reflection and Growth

What are some of your reactions after reading this chapter?

- If you're a graduate student, are you receiving comprehensive coverage of therapist–patient sexual involvement in your graduate training? If not, exploring avenues to advocate for including this area in your training could be beneficial. For those already practicing professionally, reflecting on whether this information was adequately covered during your training can shed light on potential areas for professional growth.

- How do you think having learned this information would have been helpful to you in your clinical practice? How will it be helpful now?

- Imagine yourself as a defense attorney of a famous therapist who is being sued because they engaged in sex with a patient. What arguments, justifications, excuses, rationalizations, and so forth would you make to the jury in defense of the therapist's behavior? (Feel free to make up whatever hypothetical details you like.)

- Continuing to imagine yourself as a defense attorney for a famous therapist accused of engaging in sex with a patient, how might you try to discredit the accuser?

- When you reflect on the points you made to the jury as the therapist's defense attorney, which seem like they might influence the jury? Why?

- When you reflect on your points, do you find any of them believable and inviting if you were suddenly highly attracted to a patient?

- As you review the points that you argued to the jury, do you find that you learned anything new about yourself? If so, what? And how might this knowledge affect your clinical work with clients?

3 THERAPISTS' SEXUAL FANTASIES

After providing a general introduction to this book's topics in Chapter 1 and reviewing two key aspects of sociohistorical context in Chapter 2, we now turn our attention to a topic that, with few exceptions, remains unacknowledged and unstudied in the research literature: therapists' sexual fantasies about their patients.

For such a seemingly common experience to go almost entirely unmentioned in the extensive body of psychological research raises many intriguing questions, especially the fundamental question: Why? Although we'll suggest some possible reasons that researchers have avoided the topic of therapists' sexual fantasies about their patients, we invite you to speculate on the causes now and as you read this chapter.

Sexual fantasies—defined as "any mental imagery that is sexually arousing or erotic to the individual" (Joyal, 2017, p. 1; see also Leitenberg & Henning, 1995)—can be welcome or unwanted. Some sexual fantasies may lead to joy and other pleasurable feelings while others may bring anxiety, guilt, embarrassment, confusion, or even fear that we'll be overwhelmed by the fantasy—it's power to fascinate and arouse—and do something we don't really

https://doi.org/10.1037/0000443-004
Therapists' Sexual Feelings and Fantasies: Research, Practice, Ethics, and Forensics,
by K. S. Pope, N. Y. Chavez-Dueñas, and H. Y. Adames

want to do and will regret. Some we may invoke before or during sexual activities. Others may appear unbidden at the most awkward times.

We may feel that some of our fantasies are so bizarre that no one else experiences such fantasies. However, major studies suggest that unusual sexual fantasies are rare. Examples of these statistically infrequent fantasies include sex with minors, animals, or dead human bodies and raping or engaging in other forms of sexually assaulting someone (Lehmiller & Gormezano, 2023; see also Joyal et al., 2015; Lehmiller, 2018). Research in the field of kink studies, which explores bondage and discipline, dominance and submission, and sadomasochism, has revealed that

> the prevalence of fantasies and curiosities about arousing or erotic kink activities (approximately 45–60% of the population) is much higher than the number of people who have participated in such behaviors, which can range considerably depending on region or specific behavior measured (approximately 20–46.8%). (Williams & Sprott, 2022, p. 1)

An array of fantasies that were once considered unusual—such as fetishism, frotteurism, masochism, sex in public or in a place where you might be discovered, voyeurism—turn out to be quite common (Lehmiller & Gormezano, 2023; see also Bártová et al., 2021; Joyal & Carpentier, 2017; Joyal et al., 2015; Lehmiller, 2018).

Research has uncovered group differences in sexual fantasizing. For example, several studies suggest distinct trends in sexual fantasies of people who identify as men and women. For instance, men tend to fantasize more frequently and are more likely to fantasize about scenarios involving anonymous partners and group sex (Wilson, 1997; Wilson & Lang, 1981). In contrast, women's fantasies may be more likely to feature famous people. Men and women who describe themselves as asexual are more likely to report that they have never experienced a sexual fantasy. Those who do report sexual fantasies are more likely to fantasize about sexual activities in which they were not one of the participants (Yule et al., 2017). Research also suggests that the sexual fantasies of nonbinary people are generally similar to those of cisgender individuals but are more likely to involve nonnormative genitals and less likely to represent the fantasizer as the object of desire (Lindley et al., 2020).

While it's useful to be aware of the research on group differences, it is necessary to keep in mind that these statistical patterns and trends may fail to describe a specific individual—whether ourselves, our supervisee, or one of our clients.

RESEARCH ON THERAPISTS' SEXUAL FANTASIES

The scarcity of literature on therapists' sexual fantasies can be attributed to several elements. Sociohistorical factors, such as those discussed in Chapter 2 in the section "A Freudian Start, a Watsonian Stop," may play a role. Other factors encompass the stigma associated with discussing therapists' innermost sexual experiences and how they might impact our roles as therapists. This can prompt numerous questions, including what people would think about you, how you would respond, and will you be judged?

Public Relations Problem: What Will People Think About Me?

One factor that may turn therapists away from studying therapists' sexual fantasies is apprehension regarding how colleagues and clients might perceive them. For instance, therapists may worry about clients' willingness to discuss their most sensitive and private problems with them. Therapists may also wonder if, once clients know their therapist engages in research on sexual fantasies, they might begin to question whether their therapist imagines what they looked like without clothes, fantasizes about engaging in various sexual activities with them, or uses the next break between clients to masturbate while fantasizing about them.

Curiosity About Sexual Fantasies: How Will I Respond?

Another possible reason therapists may hesitate to research therapists' sexual fantasies is unease about clients potentially inquiring about the therapist's personal sexual experiences. Clinicians may struggle with questions in this area:

- What would I say if my client directly asked about my sexual fantasies?
- What if I fantasize about my client and they ask whether I do—how would I respond?
- Would I be able to provide an ethical, therapeutic, and appropriate response?
- Would I blush and stumble over my words while thinking of how best to respond?
- How do I avoid becoming defensive?

Therapists Have Sexual Fantasies About Clients: Will I Be Judged?

Another possible cause for therapists and researchers avoiding involvement with the topic of sexual fantasies is difficulty acknowledging their own possible erotic feelings about clients and talking about them in supervision and therapy. For example, Vesentini et al. (2023) found that although most therapists believe that talking about their romantic and sexual feelings toward clients is "very important . . . only a third have disclosed their feelings in supervision, peer-supervision, or in personal therapy" (p. 263). You may wonder what the major reason is for this reluctance to disclose? The answer is the fear of being judged, shamed, or condemned.

A FREUDIAN START, A WATSONIAN STOP: WHAT CAN WE LEARN FROM THE RESEARCH?

To date, we have been unable to find any published studies that focused on therapists' sexual fantasies about clients. If we want our work to be informed by research in this area, we'll need to depend on a relatively small number of specific findings scattered across studies that address a much broader range of topics. Let's review some of these studies.

A survey of members of the American Psychological Association (APA) Division 42 (Psychologists in Independent Practice) in the mid-1980s included the question, "While engaging in sexual activity with someone other than a client, have you ever had sexual fantasies about someone who is or was a client?" (Pope et al., 1986, p. 152). Here were the results:

- almost one in five (19.3%) reported engaging in this fantasy rarely,
- 8.6% indicated that they did so occasionally,
- 0.7% reported doing so rarely,
- 71.3% reported never engaging in such fantasies about current or former clients while engaging in sex with a nonclient,
- male therapists were almost twice as likely as female therapists to report these fantasies (27% vs. 14%), and
- younger therapists were twice as likely as older therapists to report fantasies (28% vs. 14%).

The Pope et al. (1986) study of psychologists was replicated in 1994 with a national sample of clinical social workers by Bernsen and colleagues. In this study, social workers were asked the following question: "While engaging in sexual activity with someone other than a client, have you ever had sexual fantasies about someone who is or was a client?" Results indicated that

> Most therapists (78%) reported that they never had such fantasies. . . . Such fantasies were reported as occurring rarely by 15% of the therapists, often by 5%, and frequently by 1%. Male therapists were more likely to report engaging in such fantasies than were female therapists (30% vs. 13%). (p. 375)

Another study by Rodolfa et al. (1994) surveyed APA members who worked in counseling centers. They results indicated that

> Most psychologists reported that they never had sexual fantasies about former clients . . ., nor did they have sexual fantasies about current clients . . . while engaging in sexual activity with their current partner. Male psychologists reported having more sexual fantasies about clients than did female psychologists (past clients, 33% vs. 16%; current clients, 30% vs. 17%). . . . There were no differences based on age. (p. 169)

Research has also been conducted with counselors. A survey of counselors certified by the National Board for Certified Counselors indicated their beliefs about whether each of the 88 behaviors was ethical (Gibson & Pope, 1993). Notably, approximately one third (38%) expressed the view that "engaging in sexual fantasy about a client" was ethical (p. 333).

More recently, Vesentini et al. (2022) conducted a survey of 786 therapists in Flanders, Belgium. Their results highlight that "about seven out of ten therapists found a client sexually attractive [and] a quarter fantasized about a romantic relationship (22%)" (para. 1).

Research in this area can be reassuring to therapists who experience sexual fantasies about clients. These findings serve as evidence that they are not alone in this regard because a substantial portion of their peers have similarly reported such fantasies. These data also indicate that male-identifying therapists tend to report sexual fantasies about current or former clients to a significantly greater extent than therapists who identify as female. No clear patterns based on the age of therapists have emerged. Nevertheless, one study revealed that younger therapists report experiencing fantasies much more frequently than their older counterparts, while another study did not find any significant age differences (Vesentini et al., 2022).

OTHER THAN THAT, THERE'S A GAP IN KNOWLEDGE

Besides the studies and findings described in the previous section, we have no information about how therapists respond to sexual fantasies. The lack of information leaves us with many questions about this topic and how therapists make sense of these experiences, including the following:

- Do therapists enjoy having sexual fantasies about their clients?
- Do they feel ashamed or anxious about them?
- Do therapists disclose sexual fantasies to supervisors, consultants, or their own therapist?
- Do they disclose them to the client? Why or why not?

- Do they find such fantasies helpful in understanding their relationship with the client, problems or possibilities in the therapy, or other clinical issues?
- Do they feel tempted to return repeatedly to the fantasy or engage in flirtation or some form of sexualized behavior with the client?

In contrast to many other aspects of our work, in this area, we must navigate without the benefit of a wealth of studies, relying instead on scattered fragments that occasionally appear in research on other topics.

WHAT MIGHT BE HELPFUL?

It is much easier to recognize the importance of therapists' sexual fantasies when we consider our colleagues having them. It is more challenging to acknowledge that we, too, may experience them and consider how to address them openly and honestly. When experiencing sexual fantasies about a patient, it may be helpful to consider the following questions:

- Do the fantasies set off any alarm bells? In a section on "Sexual Fantasies and the Psychotherapist," Pope et al. (1984) noted that "if we begin experiencing sexual fantasies about our client, we may become alarmed and less capable of functioning therapeutically" (p. 207). If the fantasies evoke any concerns that they may impair our effectiveness as therapists, it is important that those concerns be addressed through consultation, supervision, or other resources.

- Do the fantasies put you at risk for unethical behavior?

- Do they feel potentially overwhelming, tempting you to act them out with the client, or weaken the boundaries between you and the patient?

- What resources are available to you to ensure that you do not engage in sexual behavior with the client or in other forms of sexual exploitation?

- Does experiencing sexual fantasies about the client make you feel dirty, sleazy, or like a "bad" therapist? Discussing the many myths that can afflict therapists, Pope et al. (2006) identified a particularly troublesome one: "Good therapists (i.e., those who don't sexually exploit their patients) never have sexual feelings about their patients, don't become sexually aroused during therapy sessions, don't vicariously enjoy the (sometimes) guilty pleasures of their patients' sexual experiences, and don't have sexual fantasies or dreams about their patients" (p. 28). This myth can cause deep and needless distress in good therapists.

- Do the fantasies arise from your own unmet needs—for companionship, sexual fulfillment, and so on—that should be met elsewhere (i.e., not through a client) or addressed in your own therapy?

- Do the fantasies provide any clues that might help you better understand the client, the therapeutic relationship, and the dynamics of the therapy?

Sexual fantasies involving clients are a common occurrence among therapists. These experiences may occur more often than we'd like to think about or even admit to ourselves; however, we can't address what we won't name, and we can't name what we won't openly and honestly discuss. Let's move from solely pondering about therapists' sexual fantasies to actively and purposefully exploring ways to initiate and sustain open and honest conversations on this crucial topic in our roles as scholars, therapists, supervisors, and supervisees.

4

EXPLORING POWER, SEX, GENDER, SEXUAL ORIENTATION, AND RACE IN THERAPISTS' SEXUAL FEELINGS AND FANTASIES

No matter where we go, the sum of who we are comes with us; it colors our interactions with others. Who we are perceived to be—which may be reasonably close to who we are or wildly inaccurate, depending on who is doing the perceiving—influences how other people respond—or fail to respond—to us. Power plays its part in this process. This chapter explores various sources of power, how they come into play in therapy, and how they influence therapists' sexual attraction and feelings toward patients. We pay special attention to the interplay among gender, sexuality, and race in shaping therapists' sexual attractions and fantasies.

POWER

The patient–therapist relationship involves trust and power. To echo Allen (2022), "Psychotherapy goes best when trust is reciprocal, that is, when the patient and therapist are trusting of each other and trustworthy to each other—as it should be in any close relationship" (p. xxv). To be trustworthy

https://doi.org/10.1037/0000443-005
Therapists' Sexual Feelings and Fantasies: Research, Practice, Ethics, and Forensics,
by K. S. Pope, N. Y. Chavez-Dueñas, and H. Y. Adames

in the full sense of that word (i.e., fully worthy of the patient's trust), the therapist must be aware of their power and take care to wield their influence without misusing, abusing, or exploiting the power entrusted to them by the patient, state, and profession.

Power From Our Role as Therapists

The therapist's role comes with a range of distinct powers. Consider the following seven forms of power that therapists hold (Pope et al., 2021) and their practical implications:

- power conferred by the state (e.g., engaging in actions that require a license),
- power to name and define (e.g., diagnosing a patient),
- power of testimony (e.g., testifying as an expert witness can change the course of people's lives),
- power of knowledge (e.g., understanding human behavior, mental processes, and the intrapsychic and social factors that influence people's actions),
- power of expectation (e.g., believing in the patient's ability to change),
- therapist-created power (e.g., intentionally using your power as therapist to control or influence behavior), and
- inherent power differential (e.g., having unavoidable power differences in therapy regardless of our theoretical orientation).

As therapists, we can put our power to use in the service of our patients. But we can also mishandle our power—intentionally or through carelessness or incompetence. Our power has the potential to help, heal, and enable. Misused, it can harm.

Social Group Power

Awareness of the power stemming from the social groups we are part of is critical. A *social group* refers to a collective of two or more people who are grouped together within a society on the basis of shared ideologies, socialization, and characteristics. Gender, sexual or affectional orientation,[1] race, and ethnicity are examples of social groups. The current state of the science

---

[1]"Affectional orientation expands our notion of sexual orientation. It underscores how people's attraction to others is not limited to sexuality but can also involve an emotional connection" (Pope et al., 2023, p. 78; see also Adames & Chavez-Dueñas, 2021).

seems to involve an increasing acceptance of how these categories involve social construction (see Adames, Chavez-Dueñas, & Jernigan, 2023; Allidina & Cunningham, 2023; Helms et al., 2005; Schachter et al., 2021; Smedley & Smedley, 2005; Wenzlaff et al., 2018). For example, Bonham and colleagues (2005) of the National Human Genome Research Institute, National Institutes of Health, described how different systems of racial categories were constructed and attributed to biological differences and claimed to show that some races were better than others in terms of aptitude, character, and temperament:

> Human racial classification became a focus of scientific investigation by evolutionary biologists attempting to categorize individual humans on the basis of presumed patterns of biological difference. In the 18th century, scientists hoping to categorize humans taxonomically in the same way that they categorized other species asserted that all humans belonged to four (Linnaeus, 1758) and then five (Blumenbach, 1795) groups. These scientists attached hierarchical designations to these categorizations, claiming that differences in skin color, physiognomy, and geography were associated with scientifically measurable differences in character, aptitude, and temperament (Smedley, 1998). Studies supporting these claims have since been refuted as severely flawed (Gould, 1981). Yet, in descriptions of human genetic variation, categorization of humans by "racial" and "ethnic" groups continues. Researchers must remain mindful of this historical legacy of the science of heredity as the genomic era unfolds. Current genetic data also refute the notion that races are genetically distinct human populations. (p. 12)

To take sexual orientation as another example, Katz (1995), a historian of sexuality, explained how the term *heterosexual* has evolved from its earlier origins when it was used to describe abnormal sexual practices to its contemporary understanding, noting the following:

> The earliest-known use of the word heterosexual in the United States occurs in an article by Dr. James G. Kiernan, published in a Chicago medical journal in May 1892. Heterosexual was not equated here with normal sex, but with perversion—a definitional tradition that lasted in middle-class culture into the 1920s. Kiernan linked heterosexual to one of several "abnormal manifestations of the sexual appetite"—in a list of "sexual perversions proper"—in an article on "Sexual Perversion." (p. 19)

Katz goes on to document how social forces continued to change the meaning of this term (see also Davis & Mitchell, 2021; Laqueur, 1992).

Social categories are constructed to maintain hierarchies of power. Typically, societies divide social groups into agent/dominant and target/oppressed groups. The normative standard tends to be defined by agent/dominant groups, who shape societal expectations to align with their preferences. Members of dominant groups hold higher positions in the social hierarchy, enjoying greater access to power and privilege (Harro, 2000; see also Chavez-Dueñas & Adames, 2022; Neblett et al., 2008).

Members of target or oppressed groups are placed at the lower end of the social hierarchy. They are often othered[2]—marginalized, viewed as inferior, and regarded with suspicion (Chavez-Dueñas et al., 2019). They lack access to power and experience unjust and cruel treatment in society. They may experience overlapping forms of oppressions described as intersectionality (see Adames et al., 2018; Combahee River Collective, 1995; Crenshaw, 1991; Lewis & Neville, 2015). To illustrate, heterosexual individuals typically experience more social power and privilege compared with lesbian, gay, bisexual, and queer people. However, heterosexual women may experience sexism, heterosexual Women of Color may experience not only sexism similar to White heterosexual women or racism similar to Men of Color but also a unique form of sexism that is racialized, often described as *gendered racism* (see Essed, 1991). Similarly, in many parts of the world, those born with male genitalia and features are usually granted greater access to power and more privilege compared with their siblings born with female genitalia and features, who often belong to the oppressed gender group. Trans and gender expansive People of Color have unique experiences compared with their non-People of Color counterparts.

Let's further explore these complexities, beginning with the interplay between gender and power in therapist–patient sexual involvement.

RESEARCH ON THE ROLE OF GENDER IN THERAPIST-PATIENT SEXUAL INVOLVEMENT

Research exploring therapist–patient sexual involvement has uncovered compelling findings regarding the gender of therapists who are more likely to violate ethical boundaries. In the next section, we review the research in this area.

Therapist Gender

In 1968, Bert Forer (1980), under the auspices of the Los Angeles County Psychological Association (LACPA), conducted the first survey of psychologists

---

[2]Othered or othering is described as "the process by which individuals who are perceived as 'different' [e.g., not like us, not one of us, alien, ultimately inhuman] in a given society are rejected and oppressed" (Chavez-Dueñas et al., 2019, p. 50).

to determine the rates at which members of the group reported engaging in sex with their patients. He found that 13.7% of the male psychologists and none of the female psychologists reported engaging in therapist–patient sex. However, LACPA refused to let Forer present the results publicly out of concern that the relatively high percentage of male psychologists engaging in sex with their patients would be a public relations disaster. He finally obtained approval to present the data at a 1980 meeting of the California Psychological Association.

Almost a decade later, Jean Holroyd and Annette Brodsky (1977) designed and conducted the first national survey of psychologists' sexual involvement with patients. They found that 12.1% of the male psychologists and 2.6% of the female psychologists reported having engaged in sexual activities with their patients. In 1979, Pope and colleagues conducted a subsequent national survey of psychologists with similar findings: 12.0% of male and 3.0% of female psychologists reported sexual involvement with their patients. The third national study of psychologists also included a question about engaging in sex with a former client (Pope et al., 1987). The results indicated that 3.6% of male psychologists and 0.4% of female psychologists reported engaging in sex with at least one current patient, and 14% of the male and 8% of the female psychologists reported engaging in sex with a former patient.

Lucille Gechtman and Jacqueline Bouhoutsos (1985) conducted the first national survey of social workers' sexual involvement with their clients, finding that 2.6% of male social workers and none of the female social workers reported engaging in sexual activities with their clients during therapy (see also Gechtman, 1989). The second national survey of social workers (Bernsen et al., 1994) found similar results: 3.6% of the male and 0.5% of the female social workers reported engaging in sex with a client.

Nanette Gartrell and colleagues (1986) conducted the first national survey of psychiatrists on this topic. They found that 7.1% of the male and 3.1% of the female psychiatrists acknowledged sexual contact with their patients.

A subsequent national survey sampled all three professions—1,600 psychologists, 1,600 social workers, and 1,600 psychiatrists—and found the same gender pattern emerged consistently in all the national studies: A remarkably more significant percentage of male therapists than female therapists reported engaging in sexual involvement with their clients (Borys & Pope, 1989).

Patient Gender

It will probably come as no surprise to the reader that male therapists are more likely to violate ethical standards by engaging in therapist–patient sexual involvement with female patients. The initial national study of psychiatrist–patient sex, for example, found that 88% of the "contacts for which both the psychiatrist's and the patient's gender were specified occurred between male psychiatrists and female patients" (Gartrell et al., 1986, p. 1128). In another study, Jacqueline Bouhoutsos and colleagues (1983) conducted a large survey asking therapists about any reports their clients had made to them about engaging in sexual activity with a previous therapist. They found that 92% of the reports of sex with a prior therapist involved the male therapist–female patient pattern.

A study of licensing disciplinary actions again found this trend: About 86% of the actions involving therapist–patient sex reported the therapist as male and the patient as female (Pope, 1993). The same pattern was also reflected in a survey of therapists in which a significantly higher percentage of female therapists (4.58%) than male therapists (2.19%) reported engaging in sex as patients with their therapists (Pope & Feldman-Summers, 1992).

Research in the fields of psychology, psychiatry, and social work concerning therapist–patient sexual involvement has shown a tendency for men to occupy the therapist role, while women were more likely to be patients. It is important to note that these studies were conducted in the 1970s and 1980s when a more simplistic understanding of the concepts of sex, gender, and sexuality existed.

SEX, GENDER, AND SEXUALITY

Psychology is in the midst of a slow, halting, and still incomplete journey in viewing sex, gender, and human sexuality in the simplest of terms—that is, humans are born either male or female and remain in those two dichotomous categories throughout the lifespan, and sexual and affectional orientation, a component of sexuality, is either toward one gender or the other and remains constant as long as the person lives (see Adames & Chavez-Dueñas, 2021; dickey, 2023; Morandini et al., 2021; Nakamura et al., 2022; Singh & dickey, 2017). Simultaneously, both the research and writing addressing sexual feelings in psychotherapy, as well as the distinct subject of therapist–patient sexual involvement, reflect psychology's historical position in understanding these concepts. They often lacked the depth and nuance reflective of our contemporary, more expansive perspective on sex, gender, and sexuality. Fully acknowledging, understanding, and addressing therapists' sexual feelings and therapist–patient sexual involvement is important, but it may have been hindered by (a) oversimplified and misleading definitions and theories of gender and sexual and romantic orientation and (b) leaving out the crucial context of our firsthand lived experiences of gender and sexual and affectional orientation.

Our gender and sexual and affectional orientation and how we may be oppressed because of them and other aspects of who we are influences what happens to us and how we experience those events. This context, in turn, influences how we approach, experience, understand, and address the topics of therapists' sexual feelings and therapist–patient sexual involvement. Fortunately, the field is slowly moving toward a richer, more complex, still not completely clear or settled view—or variety of views—on sex, gender, and sexuality. Before we delve further into these areas, take a moment to reflect on the following:

• What is your understanding of the meaning of "gender"?

• What factors influence or determine an individual's gender?

• What is your understanding of the meaning of "sexual orientation" or "affectional orientation"?

• What factors influence or determine an individual's sexual and affectional orientation?

• How does your understanding of these concepts and the various factors shaping them (e.g., intersecting forms of oppression) influence your perspective or comprehension of

  – a therapist sharing that they've never experienced sexual desire or attraction to a patient or anyone else;

  – a therapist who identifies as a gay male experiencing a sexual fantasy about a female patient;

  – a therapist who identifies as a heterosexual woman experiencing an intense urge to engage in sex with a female patient;

  – a therapist who describes themselves as bisexual, saying that, for some reason, they only experience sexual attraction to female (but not male) patients;

  – a therapist who identifies as a heterosexual male having an erotic dream about a male patient; and

  – a transgender therapist who says that since transitioning as an adult professional, they've ceased feeling sexually attracted to patients (but not nonpatients)?

Now that you've had an opportunity to reflect on your current understanding of the concepts of sex, gender, and sexual orientation, let's explore some themes and trends in the scientific literature.

Sex and Gender

Sex and gender are often used interchangeably but have different meanings. Scholars describe *sex* as a multidimensional biological construct based on chromosomes, reproductive organs, secondary characteristics, and hormones (National Academies of Sciences, Engineering, and Medicine, 2022; Unger, 1979). Our understanding of sex has evolved over the decades, moving away from the categorization of sex as binary (i.e., men and women) to recognize the human variations in sex differences, including intersex people (e.g., 46 XX intersex, 46 XY intersex, true gonadal intersex, complex or undetermined intersex). Currently, there are approximately 40 recognized variations categorized under intersex classifications (see Carpenter, 2018; King, 2022).

In contrast, *gender* describes sets of behaviors, traits, and expectations that a given culture associates with a person's biological sex, as described in the prior paragraph (American Psychological Association [APA], 2012; Unger, 1979). In accordance with this perspective, *gender identity* denotes an individual's internal sense of a gendered self (e.g., man, woman, male, female, womxn, agender, gender nonconforming; see Adames & Chavez-Dueñas, 2021). APA defines gender identity as "a person's deeply felt, inherent sense of being a girl, woman, or female; a boy, a man, or male; a blend of male or female; or an alternative gender" (2015, p. 834). Individuals may also be identified as cisgender or transgender. Individuals whose gender identity aligns with the genitals and biological sex characteristics they were born with are described as *cisgender*, while those who don't identify with the biological sex characteristics they were born with are described as *transgender* (American Psychological Association, 2015; Tate et al., 2014). Lastly, *gender expression* refers to how individuals communicate their gender identity through clothing, communication styles, and other actions or interests (Adames & Chavez-Dueñas, 2017).

Please take a moment to consider the following questions:

- What are some of the major ways your gender has influenced your life?

- What are three or more key ways your life might differ if you were another gender?
  - Would you have chosen a different profession?
  - Would you have been more or less successful in school?
  - Would your earnings have been different?

- Would your parents or guardians be more or less pleased with you if you were this different gender?

• Have you ever wished to be or imagined yourself as another gender?

• Have you ever experienced a sexual fantasy in which you were another gender or changed genders during the fantasy?

• Have you ever been insulted, discriminated against, or sexually or non-sexually physically attacked because of your gender expression?

Sexuality

Sexuality embodies a vital and complex dimension of human develop-ment. Sexuality encompasses our sexual attraction responses, consisting of four primary domains, including (a) *physiological*, which involves the biolog-ical response people experience in their bodies when encountering someone they find sexually attractive; (b) *affective*, which includes subjective emotional reactions an individual experiences; (c) *cognitive*, which centers on sexual thoughts, fantasies, and mental processes related to sexual attraction; and (d) *behavioral*, which pertains to the actions individuals may engage in on encountering someone they find attractive. Figure 4.1 provides a visual rep-resentation of these four components of the sexual attraction response.

Scenario

It's your day off, and you look forward to a quiet afternoon in your favorite coffee shop, drinking tea and finishing a book you've been reading. You order, sit in a cozy chair, sip your tea, and open the book. You glance up briefly and immediately lock eyes with someone you find strikingly attractive. They have just entered the coffee shop and are about to sit at the table next to yours. As your eyes meet again, a sudden "hi" from them sends a jolt through you, making your heart skip a beat. Your palms grow clammy, but you manage to say "hey" in response. When you attempt to return to your book, the words blur on the page; your mind is now elsewhere. The possibility of a conversa-tion consumes and excites you, and you start imagining embracing each other. You muster up the courage, seize the moment, and extend an invitation to share your dessert with them.

Having gone through this scenario, take a moment to reflect on the fol-lowing questions:

• Can you identify all four components of the sexual attraction response in the scenario? If not, which component(s) were more difficult to identify?

FIGURE 4.1. The Four Domains of Sexual Attraction Response

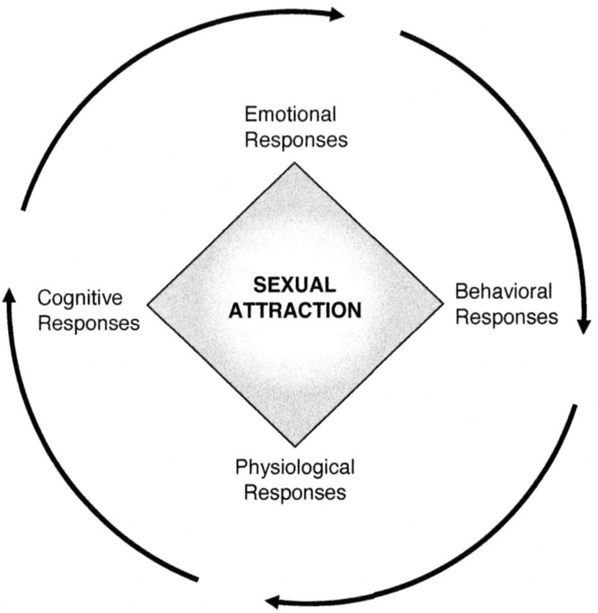

- What are some instances of physiological response?
- What are some of the emotional responses?
- In what ways was the cognitive response demonstrated in the scenario?
- Could you provide an example of a behavioral response in the scenario?

The scenario described might not completely reflect how you're inclined to react in similar situations. So, now we invite you to consider yourself in a similar situation and consider the following:

- What would you do in a similar situation?

- Take a moment to notice any physical sensations you may feel while envisioning yourself in a similar situation.

- What thoughts come to mind?

- What emotional reactions surface?

- What actions, if any, would you take?

- What actions, if any, would you like to take but refrain from taking? Why would you refrain?

- Would you share your experience and reactions with others? If so, who would that be? If not, why not?
- What if the person at the coffee shop were your client?
  - What affective, physical, emotional, and behavioral reactions will you likely experience?
  - How would you respond?

An important aspect of sexuality is sexual orientation, which is the focus of the next section. Let's keep exploring.

Sexual and Affectional Orientation

Much like our understanding of sex and gender, our understanding of sexual and affectional orientation has expanded. Currently, scholars define *sexual orientation* as "the sex of those to whom one is sexually and romantically attracted" (American Psychological Association, 2012, p. 11). Various categories exist to classify diverse sexual orientations, such as *gay* and *lesbian* for people who are attracted to members of their same sex, *heterosexual* for people who are attracted to individuals of a different sex from their own, *bisexual* for people attracted to two sexes (male and female), and *pansexuality* to describe sexual attraction to people regardless of their sex or gender (see American Psychological Association, 2012; Garnets & Kimmel, 2003; Nakamura et al., 2022; Pismenny, 2023). However, the use of distinct categories fails to capture the complexity of how sexual and affectional orientation are defined, how they exist on a continuum, and how they may be fluid for some people (Adames & Chavez-Dueñas, 2021; Diamond, 2007; Kinsey et al., 1953; Peplau & Garnets, 2000; Pope et al., 2023).

Having briefly described the typical definitions of sex, gender, and sexuality and discussed how they differ, let's explore the interplay between them. Neuroscience has advanced our understanding in this area:

> Using real-time brain scans, neuroscience research provides insight that helps us theorize about the interplay between sex, gender, gender expression, and sexual orientation. For instance, a study by Contreras et al. (2013) revealed that the first characteristics that people process when meeting others include their physiognomy (e.g., skin color, facial features) and perceived sex (Contreras et al., 2013). They describe how the brain simultaneously processes people's physiognomy and perceived sex before the person adds meaning to what they are observing. Building on this line of empirical work, we argue that when an individual comes in contact with others, they classify the person into a specific sex and make generalizations about the person's gender. However, such classification may or may not align with the person's biological sex and/or how they identify their gender. Instead, we posit that what the brain is processing is a person's gender expression which we are socialized to interpret as a person's sex and gender identity, but this may or may not be accurate. Continuing with this

thinking, we propose that people are attracted to people's gender expression, and not exclusively the person's sex or gender identity since these aspects of the self are not immediately evident to us when we encounter others. (Adames & Chavez-Dueñas, 2021, p. 63)

Why have sexual feelings in psychotherapy remained so hard for the field to fully come to terms with and address effectively? Two major reasons may be (a) oversimplified or misleading definitions and theories of gender and sexual and affectional orientation and (b) a tendency to leave out of the equation our own gender and sexual and affectional orientation, our experience(s) of them, and their effects on us and our views. Please take a moment to reflect on the following questions:

- What are some of the major ways your sexual and romantic orientation have influenced your life?

- Have you ever wished to be or imagined yourself as having a different sexual and affectional orientation?

- What are three (or more) ways your life might be different if you had another sexual or romantic orientation?
  - Would you have chosen a different profession?
  - Would you have been more or less successful in school?
  - Would your earnings have been different?
  - Would your parents or guardians be more or less pleased with you if you had this different sexual or romantic orientation?

- Have you ever been insulted, discriminated against, or sexually or non-sexually physically attacked because of your sexual or affectional orientation?

- When you find someone attractive, what specifically are you attracted to? As you think back, what assumptions did you make about the sex and gender of the people you were attracted to?

- Reflect on the people you typically find attractive; how would you describe their gender expression?

- In what ways, if any, do your gender and your sexual and affectional orientation influence your approach and role as a therapist?
  - How might they influence the clients you serve?
  - How might they influence the interventions you provide?
  - Do they influence the interactions between you and the clients you serve? If so, how?

– Can they play a role in clients that you may find attractive or have sexual fantasies about? If so, how?

RACE ALSO MATTERS IN THERAPIST-PATIENT SEXUAL INVOLVEMENT

Earlier in the chapter, we discussed the research showing that people's brains simultaneously process physiognomy (e.g., skin color, facial features, hair texture) and perceived sex when encountering a person (see Adames & Chavez-Dueñas, 2021; Contreras et al., 2013). We also described the literature on sex, gender, and sexuality in the context of therapist–patient sexual involvement. However, the prevailing body of research in this area has largely overlooked the critical role of race, which is of significant relevance in the dynamics of therapist–patient sexual involvement (see Tummala-Narra, 2021). Interestingly, like therapist–patient sexual involvement, the topic of race is often misunderstood and, when discussed, brings up discomfort, leading to the subject often being evaded (Adames, Chavez-Dueñas, & Jernigan, 2021; Helms & Cook, 1999; Neville et al., 2000), an observation that has received empirical support (see Neville et al., 2013; Sue et al., 2011; Utsey et al., 2005; Yi et al., 2023).

Revisiting Race and Racism

Race is a social construct (made up by people) created to accentuate differences derived from observable physical traits; however, race is not a biological given (Carter & Pieterse, 2005; Helms, 2008). The notion of race was created to justify *racism*, which is the interpersonal (i.e., individual acts of discrimination), cultural (i.e., devaluing the values, practices, and traditions of people who are not White), and systemic oppression (i.e., laws, policies, and practices that exclude or deny opportunities) of people based on the belief that one race is superior to another (C. P. Jones, 2000; J. M. Jones, 1972). Janet E. Helms (2008) described the connection among race, biology, and society in the context of racism:

> To say that race or racial categories are not biological designations does not mean that one's physical appearance is not biologically or genetically based. You inherited physical characteristics from your parents, and they inherited physical characteristics from your grandparents and so on. Extended family members look alike. However, White people have the power to designate which physical similarities among people are "racial," what racial label should be assigned to them, and who has the power to count categories and make

laws and policies pertaining to them. Moreover, it is the assignment of personality characteristics and behaviors to people on the basis of these factitious "racial" categories that support ongoing racism in society. (pp. 1–2)

Racialized Sexual Attraction and Fantasies

Racial dynamics are often present in our work as therapists (see Adames, Chavez-Dueñas, & Jernigan, 2023; Adames, Chavez-Dueñas, Lewis, et al., 2023; Helms & Cook, 1999; Stoute, 2020). However, therapists, even those with good intentions, often find themselves puzzled about discussing race in therapy and attending to how racism may permeate the therapeutic process. Stoute (2020) explains how:

> Historically, this subject [racial dynamic in therapy] has not been covered in clinical training programs or supervisions. It has not been addressed in clinicians' personal therapies or analyses. As a result, it is easy for therapists and patients alike to become unknowing victims of an enactment. (p. 70)

Racial dynamics may also influence a therapist's sexual attraction toward patients and how they respond to such attraction. However, a gap exists in the research concerning the process and consequences of racialized sexual attraction and fantasies within the context of therapist–patient relationships.

The few available studies on therapist–patient sexual involvement did not report the race of either the therapist or patient. Moreover, these studies were conducted in the 1970s and 1980s, a time in the field when most practitioners were White men. The question of whether a similar pattern would be observed in therapist–patient sexual involvement is an important one to investigate, especially now that the field has more People of Color and women outnumber men.

Nonetheless, there is a history of People of Color, and in particular, Women of Color, being hypersexualized and exoticized (see Brooks, 2010; Lewis et al., 2016; Mukkamala & Suyemoto, 2018). Thus, it is not difficult for us to envision these portrayals of People of Color playing out in various contexts like therapy, where there is a clear power differential between the therapist and patient.

Scenario

You are supervising a White male therapist who has been working with a young female patient of Korean descent. The patient sought help in addressing symptoms related to social anxiety. After reviewing some of their sessions' recordings, you notice the following dynamics: During the first few sessions, the client described how they felt they didn't fit in with their immigrant family and talked about wanting to be a "regular" American woman. They often made devaluing comments about people from their ethnic background and commented on how they found White people to be "so beautiful." Your supervisee smiled when this statement was made and then changed the topic.

A few sessions later, the client communicated to the therapist how much they appreciated them and how they felt comfortable talking with them. In supervision, the therapist described how proud they felt of the patient and the progress she had made in therapy. Your supervisee discussed how their patient went from having difficulty expressing their thoughts and feelings and rarely smiling to openly expressing themselves, smiling and laughing in most sessions. The supervisee also described how the client can engage socially with others outside of therapy.

More recently, you have noticed how your supervisee talks more about this patient than any of their other patients in supervision. As you watch the video recordings, you see your supervisee smiling and laughing during the session in ways you have not seen them respond to other patients.

- What are your initial thoughts and reactions to this scenario?

- How could racial dynamics potentially influence the relationship between the therapist and patient?

- How might being a woman of color influence your perception of what is taking place in the scenario?
  - How would the dynamics shift if the patient identified as a trans woman? What about if the patient was a cisgender man?
  - What about if the therapist was a man of color? Or a woman of color?

- How can the therapist's awareness of their social power, as a White man, influence their understanding of the patient's presenting concerns and their progress?

- Do you notice any patterns that may indicate the therapist is experiencing sexual attraction toward the patient?
  - If so, what indicators do you notice?
  - How would you address this with the supervisee?

In this chapter, we explored the various sources of power that often play out in therapy and discussed their connection to therapists' sexual attraction, feelings, and fantasies with patients, with an emphasis on gender, sexuality, and race. Understanding and attending to power dynamics related to gender, sexuality, and race can open pathways in therapy for us to be aware of any emotions and reactions that might arise, especially concerning the therapist's sexual attraction. This awareness enriches our professional practice while minimizing potential missteps that could adversely affect our patients.

PART II THERAPIST-PATIENT SEXUAL INVOLVEMENT

5

HOW THERAPIST–PATIENT SEX HARMS PATIENTS

A Review of the Research and Other Sources of Information

As therapists, we have an impressive range of theoretical orientations, assessment approaches, and therapeutic interventions we can draw on. Sometimes, our work may involve offering support, empathetically witnessing, and helping patients ease their distress, set aside self-defeating behaviors, achieve their goals, and live more meaningful and fulfilling lives. We do our work taking care to "do no harm."

When a therapist engages in a sexual relationship with their patient, they're setting aside the fundamental ethical responsibility to avoid doing harm and act in the client's best interest instead of the therapist's sexual impulses and desires. When therapists engage in these behaviors, they place the client at risk for profound harm. Sexual boundary violations can harm the patient, their families, the community, and the profession (Baylis, 1993; Pope et al., 2023).

In this chapter, we explore this complex and challenging topic, providing an overview of the research and other sources of information about therapist–patient sexual involvement. We focus primarily on how patients may experience harm. Acquiring a comprehensive understanding of the relevant research on the effects of therapist–patient involvement is fundamental to

https://doi.org/10.1037/0000443-006
Therapists' Sexual Feelings and Fantasies: Research, Practice, Ethics, and Forensics,
by K. S. Pope, N. Y. Chavez-Dueñas, and H. Y. Adames

51

achieving competence in this area. Awareness of the scholarship in this topic can help us to

- learn the patterns of scholarship in this area, tracing its starts and stops, resistance, misconceptions, misleading paths, and dead ends that mark its evolution;

- explore how researchers navigate issues, confront challenges, and create ways to deepen and increase our understanding about therapist–patient sexual involvement;

- enable ourselves to identify these patterns more easily so we can recognize them when they occur in our work or the work of others;

- learn about ourselves—the feelings, memories of similar occasions, and thoughts that the studies of therapist–patient sexual involvement and their findings evoke in us and how they might affect our work as therapists;

- draw on what scholarship and other sources of information have revealed about therapist–patient sexual involvement to help prepare ourselves to respond in a knowledgeable, helpful, ethical, and healing way to those who've been sexually involved with a previous therapist; and

- provide clear, well-informed testimony regarding this subject matter in depositions and trials.

KEY CONSIDERATIONS IN REVIEWING THE RESEARCH AND OTHER FORMS OF SCHOLARSHIP

As we begin, it is worth emphasizing some obvious but easily overlooked points. First, you can spend a lot of time searching for a perfect study in psychology or any other discipline and come up empty despite press releases loaded with over-the-top claims. All studies have flaws and limitations. It's important to read them with an open and sympathetic mindset—asking questions such as "What are the investigators trying to do here?" Simultaneously, maintain a critical perspective to identify any shortcomings. We can ask ourselves, "What are the errors, shortcomings, or, in more diplomatic terms, where is there room for improvement?"

Second, studies yield data, but we must use our best, most informed judgment to put those data into context. We need to see how, if at all, a study moves us forward—or blocks or misleads—in our understanding and work.

Third, all aspects must be open for thoughtful, respectful questioning and discussion. We should never hesitate to rethink a conclusion or claim, no matter how well or long the field has accepted or rejected it.

SEE NOTHING, SAY NOTHING

Therapists have historically struggled to acknowledge and discuss the issue of therapist–patient sex. Attempts to study the issue tended to meet fierce resistance. Some examples include the following:

- A therapist described urging a state professional association to study the problem and finding that some members were circulating a petition to expel them (Shepard, 1971). This is perhaps an early example of cancel culture.

- Another therapist recounted the journal rejections he received, the editors describing the issue as "too controversial" (Dahlberg, 1970, p. 34).

- Still another therapist gathered survey data for a large local professional association, but when the findings showed that a high percentage of male therapists reported engaging in sexual activities with their female patients, the board of directors ordered the researcher to set the findings aside because it was "not in the best interests of psychology to present them publicly" (see Pope & Bouhoutsos, 1986, p. 26).

The avoidance of this topic was so fierce that at one point Davidson (1977) termed it the "problem with no name" (p. 43).

Looking at the history of this topic from the vantage point of 1992, Penfold described a "conspiracy of silence" (p. 5) and identified eight factors adding to this blanket of silence:

- the belief that it only happened in the 1960s and 1970s,
- a "we–they" attitude to abusers,
- professional protectionism,
- the denial of sexual attraction to clients,
- trivialization,
- idealization of therapist–client sexual contact,
- victim-blaming, and
- the myriad fears and other feelings that hinder client disclosure (Penfold, 1992, p. 5; see also Penfold, 1998, 1999).

FINDINGS AND THEMES

As the field opened up to awareness of therapist–patient sexual involvement, investigators started gathering data about the aftermath of therapist–patient sex by interviewing patients or conducting surveys. Two pioneers in collecting these data—Phyllis Chesler and Linda Durré—set forth their conclusions in the following passages:

> Many of the women described being humiliated and frustrated by their therapists' emotional and sexual coldness or ineptitude. . . . One woman tried to kill herself; two others lapsed into a severe depression; a fourth woman's *husband*, who was also in treatment with the same therapist, killed himself shortly *after* if not *because he* found out about the affair. This particular therapist's rather sadistic and grandiose attempt to cure this woman's "frigidity" one night resulted in her developing a "headache" that wouldn't subside for a year. His behavior was depressingly typical. (Chesler, 1972, pp. 146–147)

* * *

> In my research, there were many reports of suicide attempts, severe depressions . . ., mental hospitalizations, shock treatment, and separations or divorces from husbands who just could not understand or be supportive. Women reported being fired from or having to leave their jobs because of pressure and ineffectual working habits caused by their depression, crying spells, anger, and anxiety. One woman who participated in my study eventually did commit suicide. (Durré, 1980, p. 242)

Women who successfully sued sexually exploitative therapists and wrote books about their experiences have forced the field to begin overcoming its patterns of avoidance and denial of therapist–patient sex and its effects. Pioneers such as Chesler and Durré collected data by listening to women whose therapists had engaged in sex with them. This act of listening not only increased the field's awareness of the harm resulting from therapist–patient sexual involvement but also changed the relationship between the field, which had been a passive or enabling bystander to the trauma resulting from therapist–patient sex, and the patients who'd been harmed. As Herman (2023) wrote about violence and exploitation more generally:

> The wounds of trauma are not merely those caused by the perpetrators of violence and exploitation; the actions or inactions of bystanders—all those who are complicit in or who prefer not to know about the abuse or who blame the victims—often cause even deeper wounds. These wounds are part of the social ecology of violence, in which crimes against subordinated and marginalized people are rationalized, tolerated, or rendered invisible. (p. 3)

In the context of "the problem with no name" and the conspiracy of silence, the seemingly simple and reasonable act of listening became, in Herman's words, "a radical act" (2023, p. 9).

As reports and studies of harm accumulated, two major themes began to emerge: (a) the similarity of therapist–patient sex to the trauma of rape and (b) the harmful impact akin to that of incest. Masters and Johnson's (1976) research made an impact in part because of the large number of participants in their research. Their data led them to conclude that

> when sexual seduction of patients can be firmly established by due legal process, regardless of whether the seduction was initiated by the patient or the therapist, the therapist should be sued for rape . . . i.e., the legal process should be criminal. (p. 3371; see also Masters & Johnson, 1966, 1970)

Finkelhor (1984) agreed with Masters and Johnson that patient consent never justified therapist–patient sex but compared the sexual involvement with incest because of "the fundamental asymmetry of the relationship. A patient. . . cannot freely consent to sex with a therapist" (Finkelhor, 1984, p. 18). Subsequently, a broad and diverse array of researchers and others focusing on this area has discussed how the dynamics and other aspects of therapist–patient sex resemble those of rape and incest (see Pope, 1990b).

Some therapists tried to blame the victim by claiming it was the patient's fault, that patients had asked for it, worn provocative clothing, seduced the therapist, fallen in love with the therapist, and so on. These attempts to avoid responsibilities were rejected by the profession. Gutheil and Gabbard (1992) wrote:

> Clinicians knowledgeable in this area are well aware that a significant fraction of sexual misconduct instances are initiated by the patient. Such initiation empirically encompasses the full realm of human interaction from innuendo to overt requests, demands, threats, and blackmail, even to the threat of suicide. . . . Subject to no code, patients are free to demand, request, and threaten as they wish. These behaviors are suitable for therapeutic exploration; the therapist alone bears the blame for acting on these behaviors, since axiomatically only the therapist can be blameworthy. (p. 518; see also Alpert & Steinberg, 2017; Baylis, 1993; Folman, 1991; Gabbard, 1991; Nugent, 1994; Penfold, 1987; Pope, 1988, 1990a, 1990b; Simon, 1999)

METHODS AND PERSPECTIVES

The pioneering research studies on how therapist–patient sexual involvement affects patients became a cascade (e.g., Ben-Ari & Somei, 2004; Bouhoutsos et al., 1983; L. S. Brown, 1988; Butler & Zelen, 1977; Feldman-Summers &

Jones, 1984; Herman et al., 1987; Nachmani & Somer, 2007; Pope & Vetter, 1991; Somer & Saadon, 1999; Sonne & Jochai, 2014; Sonne et al., 1985; Vinson, 1987). Our understanding of the effects of therapist–patient sexual involvement draws not only from civil and criminal cases and patients' first-hand accounts in articles and books but also from an array of studies using standardized psychological assessment instruments, clinical interviews, and behavioral observations.

Studies have included patients who began subsequent therapy, as well as those who never returned to therapy. Effects have been evaluated by

- the patients themselves,
- independent clinicians, and
- subsequent therapists (for those patients who sought additional therapy).

Consequences for patients who were sexually involved with a therapist have been compared with those for matched groups of (a) therapy patients who have not been sexually involved with a therapist and (b) patients who have been sexually involved with a (nontherapist) physician (Pope, 1992; Pope & Bouhoutsos, 1986).

The accumulated scholarship, taken as a whole, makes it difficult to avoid concluding that, ethical and legal issues aside, a therapist who decides to engage in sexual activities with a patient is knowingly and intentionally deciding to place that patient at risk for significant harm. As Martin and Beaulieu (2023) wrote in their 20-year review of cases in Quebec, "The sexualization of the professional relationship is considered especially serious as it is associated with a strong potential for harm" (para. 2).

EFFECTS ON OTHERS

Gómez et al. (2021) discussed a therapist's decision to engage in sex with a patient as an act of betrayal, often resulting in betrayal trauma. They emphasized that the therapist is betraying not only the patient but also their colleagues, with the effects of "colleague betrayal" initially coined and described by Courtois (2017, p. 251). Consider how you feel when you learn that a colleague has engaged in sex with a patient. How, if at all, does it matter

- if you referred the patient to that therapist?
- if that therapist is a member of your clinic, your group practice, or the psychology department at your university or professional school?
- if that therapist is or was your supervisor?
- if that patient is your best friend?
- if that patient is your son or daughter?
- if that patient is your spouse or partner?

- if that patient identified as a woman?
- if that patient identified as a man?
- if that patient identified as transgender?
- if that patient identified as a lesbian, gay, or bisexual person?
- if that patient was a person of color?

Consider how that might affect the patient's family and friends. Think about how it might affect those who taught, supervised, and licensed the therapist. Consider how it might model behavior for students and fellow professionals. Consider how it might affect people who are in therapy or considering seeking help from a therapist. Consider how it might affect policymakers.

Having started to engage actively with the issues through questions, we provide an opportunity to engage in an activity for self-reflection and growth.

AN INVITATION FOR SELF-REFLECTION AND GROWTH

One significant hurdle in recognizing, acknowledging, and openly discussing issues related to therapist–patient sexual involvement is the divisive we–they attitude that often exists concerning therapists engaging in this behavior (Penfold, 1992). We invite you to consider the following questions:

- Where, if at all, do you see the we–they tendency in yourself?
- If you see a tendency to treat such therapists as "other," what might cause, nurture, or reinforce that mindset?
- What strategies can you identify that might assist you in overcoming a we–they tendency?
- What other, if any, of Penfold's eight barriers do you see in yourself?
- What are the causes, strengtheners, or reinforcers of these barriers?
- How might they be overcome?

In this chapter, we discussed the potential harm to patients resulting from therapist–patient sexual involvement, an area that often doesn't receive much attention within and outside the field. We invite you to reflect on the following prompts:

- How were these issues discussed during your graduate training, if at all?
- If the information in this chapter is new to you, what thoughts and reactions did you have as you were reading?
- How might you apply the knowledge acquired about the negative impact of therapist–patient sexual involvement to enhance your role as a therapist?
- What makes integrating this knowledge important to our clinical work?
- What are the barriers—psychological, social, cultural, professional, or otherwise—to acquiring, integrating, and applying this knowledge?

6 THERAPIST VULNERABILITIES

Why do some therapists engage in sexual behaviors with their patients? Why and how do they start inching, however slowly, toward starting sexual activities with a patient? Or why do they lurch suddenly into sexual involvement?

We know what is at stake. Crossing that bright line violates an ancient ethical prohibition and the current professional ethical code. We know it breaks legal and professional standards. As the studies reviewed earlier in this book made clear, it puts clients at risk for significant and lasting harm. It places the therapist at risk for loss of reputation, work, and license; opens them up to a malpractice suit; and, in some jurisdictions, risks loss of liberty through criminal convictions. So why are some therapists—including some of the most prominent and influential leaders in the field (see Chapter 2)—willing to roll the dice with their patients' safety and well-being and their own integrity, ethics, license, and so much else?

In this chapter, we'll explore these questions and set aside tendencies to dismiss therapists who engage in sex with patients as an alien group of "others" completely unlike us, whose motivations, self-talk, and decision making remain at a safe distance, a murky mystery having nothing to do with any of us who would never even consider crossing that line. What might make

https://doi.org/10.1037/0000443-007
Therapists' Sexual Feelings and Fantasies: Research, Practice, Ethics, and Forensics,
by K. S. Pope, N. Y. Chavez-Dueñas, and H. Y. Adames

us vulnerable to making bad—perhaps terrible—decisions in this area or ease the way downward? In the following sections, we present and describe eight common factors.

POWERFUL, PERSISTENT, OR INDULGED FANTASIES

Sexual attraction to a client is a common occurrence, and sometimes, a sexual fantasy will accompany that attraction. However, if the fantasy is powerful, persistent, or indulged, it may tempt the therapist to act on it and make it real. Powerful sexual fantasies can evoke instant, intense sexual arousal, making it difficult not to engage in some form of sexual behavior. They may be intrusive and come unbidden at the most awkward and inappropriate times, perhaps when we are most vulnerable.

Persistent sexual fantasies don't simply pass through the therapist's awareness but seem to set up residence in the mind, constantly returning to awareness. Indulged fantasies are those that are actively nourished, making them more elaborate, vivid, and detailed as the therapist enjoys them, perhaps calling up the images or narrative during masturbation or sexual behavior with another individual.

What is important when experiencing powerful, persistent, or indulged sexual fantasies about a client is to recognize that it may reflect a growing vulnerability and it is an issue that needs attention. In some instances, the therapist may be able to sort through what's happening on their own; in others, consultation, supervision, or therapy may be helpful. During this process of sorting through or getting help from others, therapists should be especially alert for rationalizations, such as the highly unlikely proposition that the therapeutic relationship will be either helped or completely unaffected by the therapist fantasizing about sexual intercourse or other sexual behavior with the client.

LONELINESS

Loneliness can make us vulnerable to violating important boundaries, including having sex with clients. Suppose we are lonely and grappling with shyness, finding it hard to make friends, and lacking deep and fulfilling relationships that nourish us. Our vulnerability and unfilled needs in this area may lead us to try to fulfill these yearnings with a psychotherapy patient. In therapy, we may have someone we find attractive right in front of us. Someone with whom we might already be talking about important things in their life.

That conversation might be subtly, gradually turned toward more romantic or sexual territory when this content is not part of the patient's treatment. The patient might, supposedly as a part of the therapy and following your lead, be encouraged to talk about the topic. Perhaps you guide the conversation in such a way that it makes it more likely that the patient will become aroused while remembering, imagining, or discussing something sexual and related topics. Examples include the following:

- asking them to recall their first sexual experience (or first orgasm, first experience masturbating, etc.) and then discuss it;
- asking them to describe what turns them on;
- asking them to describe some of their sexual fantasies;
- asking them if they ever became sexually aroused when it was surprising, inappropriate, or unwanted—then discussing the dynamics;
- asking what aspects of sex make them feel ashamed or embarrassed;
- asking them if there are aspects of their sexuality that they are uneasy, confused, conflicted, or concerned about;
- asking them if they've ever read or watched pornography and, if so, to describe the pornography and their reaction to it;
- asking them if they ever felt so aroused that they felt out of control;
- asking them what, if any, fantasies they experience during masturbation or sex with other people; and
- asking them to describe in as much detail as possible what they experience physically when they masturbate.

Putting all these questions together in a list makes it clear how harshly intrusive and clumsily manipulative they are and how they serve the therapist's desires rather than the healing and welfare of the patient or the goals of a legitimate treatment plan. However, when a single question or suggestion is tailored to an individual patient's history, needs, vulnerability, or transference and eased into the discussion, it may blend in with the therapeutic context and draw on the patient's trust, compliance, determination to work hard in therapy even when uncomfortable, and desire to please the therapist.

Therapists may cleverly present selfish and inappropriate questions or suggestions in the guise of

- discovering whatever seems to be getting in the way of the client being at ease during sex and experiencing orgasms or experiencing them more easily or intensely;

- understanding how formative events in the client's history shaped their sexuality and resulted in unresolved difficulties related to the issues that brought them to therapy—somewhat more challenging to sell if the patient's presenting problem is sesquipedalophobia (fear of long words), octophobia (fear of the number eight), or kinemortophobia (fear of zombies—which, to the authors of this book, seems a fairly reasonable thing to be afraid of);

• understanding a complex network of dynamics that may be at the heart of why the client might have been frustrated in trying to form a deep, lasting, meaningful, and fulfilling romantic partnership;

• helping clients understand their negative self-concept and difficulty with true self-acceptance when it comes to their bodies;

• empowering clients to reach, welcome, and unleash the miraculous energy that remains frustratingly bottled up and that redirects itself into negative, self-defeating behaviors, anxiety, and depression;

• empowering clients to embrace confidence and be more open in talking about sexuality, which can help them develop stronger connections with sexual partners; and

• revealing thoughts, emotions, experiences, and memories that have been repressed, suppressed, blocked, or distorted in a way that keeps profound aspects of clients' authentic selves perpetually concealed. This can lead to a sense of self-perplexity and a lack of understanding about their inner world and direction—a state of feeling lost, unfulfilled, not on the right path, and not living the life they want to live.

Readers can probably add to this list of cons.

Experiencing loneliness as a therapist does not, of course, automatically lead every clinician to manipulate and exploit their clients for their own benefit. However, being lonely means that we have to pause and consider how this experience may affect our clinical work. Recognizing that loneliness can lead to counterproductive situations in our work with clients, we can better prepare ourselves by seeking emotional, physical, and sexual connection with individuals we do not oversee, treat, or have power over in ethical and life-affirming ways. In our work as therapists, we must remain aware that loneliness often—though not always—goes hand in hand with isolation.

ISOLATION

Isolation is often related to loneliness, but not always. Consider people who feel most lonely when they are at a party. Isolation can create a unique form of vulnerability, often going unnoticed and different from the susceptibility resulting from loneliness. Our work as therapists can be isolating. Most of us work with individuals, but even those who work with couples, families, or groups can spend virtually our whole day with patients, isolated from the casual give-and-take we have with our family, friends, and even friendly acquaintances. We cannot—or should not—look to our patients to meet our social and emotional needs and our desires for physical touch and connection.

If we are in solo practice, we may lack even the quick "hellos" and small talk with clinicians, administrators, and other employees that are routine in clinics, hospitals, community mental health centers, and similar organizations. We might not always have someone available to share our work-related excitement and frustrations with and to provide us with affirmation and support. The private office, isolated from shared receptionists, waiting areas, and so on, can also offer the kind of extreme privacy that can make us believe that sexual engagements with a patient are less likely to be discovered. Experiencing isolation can also arise when working for an agency delivering services remotely via telehealth. In such situations, we may find ourselves working from home or a remote setting, devoid of the tangible and emotional connections present in face-to-face mental health agencies.

NEEDINESS

Virtually all of us go through periods when we are especially needy. Sometimes, this neediness follows the breakup of a significant relationship, a crisis of faith, the passing of a loved one, a physical trauma, a professional disappointment, an existential crisis, or countless other causes. Other times, there is no apparent cause, and a sense of extreme neediness suddenly catches us off guard, seeming to come out of nowhere. This neediness can make us vulnerable to heading down slippery slopes toward bad decisions.

Among the first to identify neediness as a risk factor for therapists who engage in sex with clients was Dahlberg (1970). Examining nine instances of therapist–patient sexual involvement, he concluded, "People who have some unfilled need are more likely to succumb to temptation" (p. 118). In their 1977 study, Butler and Zelen examined 20 psychiatrists and psychologists who had engaged in sexual activities with their patients. Echoing Dahlberg's pioneering work, they wrote: "One might assume the therapists shifted their sources of gratification to their patients during these vulnerable or needy periods of time" (p. 142). Discussing therapists who engage in sex with patients, Smith (1989) similarly referred to

> a profound need for reassurance. . . . Under such circumstances these thera-
> pists usually abandon the psychotherapy processes to confide their personal

problems to the patient, which may then arouse the patient to find ways to comfort the therapist, and this comfort can be quickly turned into sexual acts. (p. 61)

More recently, Strean's (2018) study resulted in this formulation:

It would appear that just as the patient who feels injured and needs care can fall in love with a therapist and want to have sex, the therapist who engages in sex with his patient feels just as wounded and just as needy. (p. 28)

In discussing neediness and other vulnerabilities in this context, it is important to emphasize that these are normal, human experiences quite common among therapists. If we are feeling a little "out there" and alone in terms of this or that vulnerability, it is good to remind ourselves that, as Harry Stack Sullivan (1947) wrote, "We are all much more simply human than otherwise" (p. 7). Recognizing that we all have needs and can, at times, feel needy is an essential first step. It is also important to become aware of how these experiences could affect our work.

Awareness of our vulnerabilities and how we typically respond to them is critical but is not a good reason to feel anxious or concerned about the vulnerability. We can experience our vulnerabilities and continue to work safely, ethically, and competently. Suppose we are distressed by a feeling of vulnerability or being overwhelmed, unable to function well, or at risk in any way. In that case, it's time to take immediate steps to find help, support, and guidance. In extreme instances, we may need to step away temporarily from our work with patients. In most cases, however, we can continue to do good work while being aware of our vulnerabilities. As Winnicott (1965) wrote, "The psychotherapist . . . must remain vulnerable and yet retain [their] professional role in [their] actual working hours" (p. 160).

A SENSE OF GRANDIOSITY AND SELF-CENTEREDNESS

Experiencing a sense of overconfidence, such as believing that we alone can heal our patients and fix what is wrong with them, is another potential risk factor. Here, we are not talking about formal personality disorders or diagnosable mental problems but rather either enduring traits or more temporary states. We are describing how we may feel super powerful and effective, at least in terms of the patient we will become sexually involved with. We may think we completely understand them and their problems in a way no one else could. We bask and luxuriate in our remarkable skills as we put them to use in this situation. Slowly and subtly, we may inadvertently shift our focus away from addressing the client's presenting concerns and develop an inappropriate romantic or sexual relationship with them. Although we may find excitement, pleasure, and joy in thinking about and being with our new sexual and romantic companion, our focus has subtly shifted from the patient and the patient's needs to ourselves, our needs, our powers and skills, our unique role in the patient's life, and our newfound pleasure.

Jehu (1994) was among the first to identify this pattern among many therapists who engage in sex with their patients. He wrote,

> Such therapists feel competent and entitled to use unorthodox therapeutic approaches—perhaps including sexual contact—which are beyond the more limited powers of lesser therapists. Being overconfident in themselves, they do not deign to seek help or advice from others. Very often patients perceive them as charismatic gurus. (p. 62)

Often, this grandiose feeling that we alone can help this patient fits neatly into the role of rescuer, which can bring its own cascade of cruel consequences.

> Perhaps the most difficult trap to avoid is the feeling that one is indispensable, that only through personal intervention can one provide a patient with the feeling that he or she is [or they are] lovable, desirable, or worthwhile. Rescuers in the helping professions are particularly prone to encourage attenuated dependency on the therapist and to discourage social networks, a reversal of the healing process. (Pope & Bouhoutsos, 1986, p. 45)

CHARACTER DISORDERS WITH IMPULSE CONTROL

A special subset of therapists who engage in sexual misconduct with clients has been identified in the literature. As an example, Schoener and Gonsiorek (1988) conducted groundbreaking research, examining more than 1,000 cases of therapist–patient sex. Their findings indicated that therapists in such cases often exhibited characteristics such as cunning, calculating behavior, emotional detachment, and a smooth demeanor. Their expertise is seducing a large and diverse array of patients while avoiding detection. They range from low-profile, obscure therapists who are relatively unknown and unnoticed in the professional community to prominent, highly accomplished, award-winning leaders (see Chapter 5). Schoener and Gonsiorek wrote,

> This group is adept at manipulating others. There is usually a long string of victims (sometimes well-hidden), who range from clients to other professionals, third-party payers, and so on. Through manipulation and/or well-timed threats, these perpetrators often induce clients, colleagues, and professional organizations to help them avoid the consequences of their misdeeds. When caught, they often do a remarkable job of mimicking a healthy therapist who

is remorseful and confesses to things that they believe are already known. . . . Although some in this group will voluntarily seek therapy and appear to be involved in a rehabilitation effort, they are not candidates for change. (p. 67)

THERAPISTS WHO BECOME SEXUALLY INVOLVED WITH CHILDREN

Some therapists may not only engage in sexual relationships with adult clients but also abuse their power by sexually exploiting children and adolescents. A survey of psychologists published in *American Psychologist* found that around 24% reported that they had encountered instances of sexual involvement between therapists and minor patients (Bajt & Pope, 1989). Approximately 56% of the minor patients were female, spanning an age range of 3 to 17 years, with an average age of approximately 14. The age of the minor male patients ranged from 7 to 16, with a mean of roughly 12.

Further information about therapist–patient sex involving minors emerged from a national survey of 1,320 psychologists in which about half of the respondents reported assessing or treating at least one patient who had engaged in sexual activities with a previous therapist, for a total of 958 such cases (Pope & Vetter, 1991; see also Capawana, 2016; Waisman, 2017). In about 5% of these cases, the patient was a minor at the time of the sexual activities with their therapist. While there are some data about therapists engaging in sex with minors, more information is needed to help us identify the patterns and risk factors that may be unique to individuals in this category.

GENDER

Perhaps the earliest identified therapist factor associated with therapist–patient sexual involvement was gender. Research indicates that a higher percentage of therapists who identify as men compared with therapists who identify as women become sexually involved with their patients. In the first national survey of therapist–patient sex, Holroyd and Brodsky (1977) found that 10.9% of licensed psychologist men and 1.9% of the licensed psychologist women reported engaging in erotic contact with their therapy patients. The researchers concluded that their findings suggested that

three professional issues remain to be addressed: (a) that male therapists are most often involved, (b) that female patients are most often the objects, and (c) that therapists who disregard the sexual boundary once are likely to repeat.

The concern of feminist psychologists (Chesler, 1971; Hare-Mustin, 1974; Henley, 1971) and of the APA Task Force on Sex Bias and Sex Role Stereotyping in Psychotherapeutic Practice (American Psychological Association, 1975) that erotic contact with patients is based on therapist needs for power or sexual gratification seems justified. (Holroyd & Brodsky, 1977, p. 849)

The eight national studies that were published over the next 17 years, surveying a total of 5,148 psychologists, psychiatrists, and social workers, found that an average of 6.8% of the male therapists and 1.6% of the female therapists reported having engaged in sexual activities with at least one patient (Akamatsu, 1988; Bernsen et al., 1994; Borys & Pope, 1989; Gartrell et al., 1986; Holroyd & Brodsky, 1977; Pope et al., 1979, 1986, 1987). More recently, Pope et al. (2021) provided a review of these and other data sources about gender and therapist–patient sexual involvement.

These and subsequent studies of gender have tended to focus our attention on the major pattern of male therapists engaging in sexual activities with female patients. However, in a section titled "Minorities Masked by the Majority," Pope (1994) emphasized that "one unfortunate consequence of this stark gender pattern is that it has contributed to the smothering of adequate attention to the relatively small minority that involves other dyads (such as woman–woman or man–man), triads, or larger groups" (p. 19).

INVITATION FOR SELF-REFLECTION AND GROWTH

Virtually all the people reading this book likely think that they would never choose to become sexually involved with a client. However, the data suggest that a small minority do, and none of us is free from vulnerabilities. So, as you finish reading this chapter, we invite you to consider the following:

- How many of your vulnerabilities can you identify, even if they were not mentioned in this chapter and even if you are confident that they could never mark the start of a journey that would include engaging in sex with a patient?

- What thoughts or emotions do you have as you identify each one? Are any of them painful or otherwise difficult to think about? Are you ashamed of any of them?

- Which of these have you disclosed to at least one other person? Have you kept any of them completely secret?

- Take a moment to consider what it feels like to recognize that you, too, have some vulnerabilities that have been identified as risk factors for engaging in sexual relationships with clients.

- What steps could you take to address each of those vulnerabilities, even if you doubted the steps were necessary?

- Even if you cannot identify any vulnerabilities in the present, what new vulnerabilities can you anticipate reasonably experiencing in the future? For example, most of us will experience at least one devastating event, such as a deep betrayal, divorce, life-threatening illness, death of a loved one, disabling trauma, or financial catastrophe during our career.

- What steps could you take to address each of those vulnerabilities should you run into them sometime during your career?

- Suppose you were to experience sexual attraction to a client and were at serious risk for engaging in some form of sexual activity with them. What resources would be most helpful and effective in pulling you back from the cliff? How can you plan to ensure you have these resources available if you ever need them?

PART **III** FORENSIC COMPETENCE

7

REACTIONS, BIASES, AND THE BASICS OF PARTICIPATING IN FORENSIC WORK INVOLVING THERAPIST–PATIENT SEX

In forensic work, therapists put their clinical expertise to work, helping individuals and institutions navigate legal matters. Some therapists specialize in forensic work, qualifying to testify as *expert witnesses* and to give their expert professional opinions. Others testify as *fact witnesses*, limiting their testimony to describing the basic facts they know firsthand about their treatment of a client. Both fact and expert witnesses can testify in cases where therapist–patient sexual involvement is alleged. In these cases, therapists may enter the realm of forensic work through diverse paths, including the following:

- testifying as a fact witness about a current or former client who is suing another therapist, alleging therapist–patient sexual involvement;

- testifying as a fact witness about a current or former client who is a therapist and is being sued by a former client of theirs, alleging therapist–patient sexual involvement;

- submitting a forensic report about a current or former client involved in a licensing board hearing involving allegations of therapist–patient sexual involvement;

https://doi.org/10.1037/0000443-008
Therapists' Sexual Feelings and Fantasies: Research, Practice, Ethics, and Forensics,
by K. S. Pope, N. Y. Chavez-Dueñas, and H. Y. Adames

- testifying as an expert witness in a licensing board hearing involving allegations of therapist–patient sex;

- testifying as a fact witness about a current or former client who is either a defendant or a witness for the prosecution in a criminal trial focusing on allegations of therapist–patient sexual involvement;

- testifying as an expert witness in a criminal trial focusing on allegations of therapist–patient sexual involvement; and

- testifying as a defendant in a licensing board hearing, civil litigation, or criminal trial involving allegations of therapist–patient sexual misconduct.

These and other paths to forensic work take us from the familiar world of psychotherapy into a different world with its own set of rules, assumptions, and approaches. In this chapter, we describe the different rules and expectations for therapists when working with clients on issues related to therapist–patient sexual involvement in a clinical versus forensic setting.

DIFFERENT WORLDS

Psychotherapy and forensic work involve distinct practices, processes, and goals. In therapy, the therapist and client usually work together toward mutually agreed-on goals. These goals and the interventions used to reach them are typically reflected in the informed consent process provided before the beginning of treatment. Alternatively, forensic work occurs in an adversarial system, pitting attorneys and litigants against each other. In treatment, the therapist decides what to say; in court, the judge decides what testimony is admissible. In therapy, the therapist usually—but with important exceptions—chooses what to say based on what is in the client's best interest. In court, the therapist takes an oath to tell the truth, the whole truth, and nothing but the truth, regardless of whether the truth helps or hurts anyone's interests, including the client's. What is said and done in therapy is usually confidential. What is said and done in court usually becomes part of the public record, available to anyone, including the media.

Forensic work is a vast array of different worlds. Licensing and other administrative hearings, civil courts in which malpractice and other suits are tried, and criminal courts have different rules and procedures. Federal courts have different rules and procedures from state and provincial courts, and each state and province has unique rules and procedures. U.S. courts differ significantly from Canadian and other countries' courts.

Before heading into a new forensic world within a specific jurisdiction, we need to consider the specific rules and procedures that will govern our work:

- Will our work for an attorney be treated as confidential and privileged "work product," or will our reports be subject to subpoena? Can we be subpoenaed to testify in court?

- If we are testifying, will it be as a fact witness or expert witness? A fact witness can usually report only what they have personally experienced through the five senses. An expert witness can make inferences, draw conclusions, and express professional opinions.

- Does our licensing status meet the criteria for doing forensic work in the relevant jurisdiction?

- Does our professional liability insurance cover forensic work in the relevant jurisdiction?

REACTIONS

Earlier sections of this book explored how our sexual attractions to clients often make us uncomfortable, sometimes evoking guilt, anxiety, and confusion. After understanding the sharp differences between the clinical and forensic realms, the second key to effective forensic work is realizing how these emotional reactions, especially if unacknowledged, can complicate and undermine our forensic work in this area. The range of emotional reactions can, if not recognized and addressed, sabotage forensic work, particularly in cases involving allegations of therapist–patient sex. Here are a few examples:

- We may overidentify with the client and want to avenge the wrongs they are alleging, resulting in our exaggerating the harm attributed to the therapist–patient sex.

- We may overidentify with the accused therapist, focusing our report and testimony on discrediting the client and painting an idealized portrait of the therapist.

- If we are sexually attracted to the therapist or client, we may slant our work to favor that person.

- If we are strongly attracted to someone involved in the case, our frustration and not being able to pursue a sexual relationship immediately may cloud our judgment and work.

- If we have viewed ourselves as happy and fulfilled in a monogamous relationship, our strong attraction to someone involved in the case may throw us off stride and interfere with our work. For instance, if we identify as exclusively heterosexual males or lesbians and find ourselves attracted to or fantasizing about a male litigant, these feelings and fantasies may be disorienting and impact our professional judgment. The attraction and fantasies may have a disorienting effect and cloud our work. Readers can supply the other seeming mismatches.

- If we find ourselves experiencing powerful, persistent, or indulged sexual fantasies about someone involved in the case, it may make it difficult to concentrate and think clearly about our work.

- If our sexual feelings about someone involved in the case make us feel anxious, guilty, ashamed, disappointed in ourselves, and reluctant to acknowledge and examine our feelings, these feelings may find expression in our work, undermining the integrity, fairness, and validity of our conclusions and testimony.

There is no one-size-fits-all set of steps to acknowledging and addressing such reactions in a way that will support—or at least not undermine—our work. To some degree, it will depend on our theoretical orientation: Cognitive behavior, psychoanalytic, existential, feminist, decolonial, interpersonal, acceptance and commitment, multicultural, dialectical behavioral, liberation, family systems, and narrative therapists are likely to have different approaches and other vocabularies for describing those approaches.

When you're stuck, ask yourself, "What do I least want to do?" and consider doing that. This could mean stepping away for some alone time, confiding in a trusted colleague or supervisor, seeking professional guidance, or anything else that feels right. The key is to keep exploring options until you're confident you're honest with yourself and effectively addressing the situation. This approach can be particularly helpful when you suspect you know the right course of action, but your mind is resisting it. By confronting your avoidance, you may bring the solution into clearer focus.

The emotional reactions may not be evoked by something directly related to the therapist–patient sexual involvement. Consider whether each of the following might affect your forensic work on a case involving therapist–patient sex and how you might handle the situation.

BIASES

Another vital aspect of meeting and upholding the highest standards in engaging in therapist–patient sex forensic work involves carefully becoming aware of and addressing our biases. The process begins with recognizing that all of us—along with our instruments, approaches, and judgments—lack perfection. We make mistakes. Our assessment instruments and methods are not flawless in terms of validity, reliability, and applicability. Our reports sometimes fail to capture the nuances of our conclusions accurately; the data on which they are based; important information we did not have access to, overlooked, or chose to omit; and our reservations. The reports are often subject to—and sometimes invite—misinterpretations.

When these flaws are random, they are termed *noise* (Kahneman et al., 2021). However, they show bias when they systematically veer in one direction over another. For example, a therapist whose client's attorney calls them to testify in the client's lawsuit against a previous therapist may find themselves shading their testimony to hide any information that might hurt the client's case. A therapist who wants to start a forensic practice and is having a hard time meeting expenses might feel a strong pull toward delivering reports that they believe will please the attorney who hired them and lead to additional business. Some of us may instinctively or through prior experiences identify with defendants, others with plaintiffs. When called to testify as expert witnesses, our testimony may be biased toward the side we identify with. Recognizing the factors that can shape our tendency or difficulty identifying with a litigant is crucial. Some of the many factors that might affect the degree to which we do or don't identify with a specific litigant include the person's race, gender, sexual orientation, weight, affect, politics, religion, income, clothing, accent, or disability.

Some experts make a career out of testifying as expert witnesses for just the defense, just the prosecution, or just the plaintiff. They become the go-to person for attorneys looking for a reliable expert and, unless crumbling in the face of an especially effective cross-examination, rarely disappoint the attorney who hired them. They will likely see always testifying for one side as effective specialization; others will see it as bias.

Confirmation Bias

A human bias that tends to influence many of us is *confirmation bias,* artfully described in 1620 by Francis Bacon (1955):

> The human understanding when it has once adopted an opinion . . . draws all things else to support and agree with it. And though there be a greater number

and weight of instances to be found on the other side, yet these it either neglects or despises, or else by some distinction sets aside and rejects. . . . This mischief insinuates[s] itself into philosophy and the sciences; in which the first conclusion colors and brings into conformity with itself all that come after. (p. 472)

We may start a forensic assessment with the idea that the person we're evaluating is dishonest, mentally impaired, or suffering from borderline personality based on social group membership biases, first impressions, what an attorney told us, or a clinical case report from a decade ago. It may be extremely difficult not to allow this idea to guide our assessment, conclusions, report, and testimony. Brodsky (2023) noted that bias can harden into stubbornness:

Stubbornness is a particularly obvious example of confirmation bias. . . . Confirmation bias causes people to attend systematically to evidence that supports their opinion and to reject evidence that disproves it. When this happens on the stand, it can be obvious to everyone in the courtroom, except the stubborn expert. The unwillingness to yield on any point, even one that seems obviously true, decreases the expert's credibility in the eyes of the triers of fact. (p. 26)

Correspondence Bias

In forensic assessment and testimony, *correspondence bias*, also known as the *fundamental attributional error* (Ross, 1977; see also Ross, 2018), emphasizes an individual's attitudes, character, and personality while paying little attention to or ignoring entirely situational factors. This bias causes us to downplay our own "bad" behavior as caused by the situation (i.e., it's not our fault) while attributing similar lousy behavior of others to who they are as a person. We can't produce the subpoenaed clinical records because we just moved offices, our computer crashed, destroying those files, and our secretary forgot to make backups. However, the person we're evaluating cannot produce files that were subpoenaed because they are dishonest, they likely hid or purposely destroyed the files, and they have criminal tendencies.

Racial Bias

A third common form of bias is *racial bias*. It is crucial to understand how racial bias—both subtle and obvious—can affect not only our attitudes and judgments but also our methods and instruments. The original Minnesota Multiphasic Personality Inventory (MMPI; Hathaway & McKinley, 1943) provides a stark example. The original MMPI and its revised versions have been the most widely used forensic instruments (Pope et al., 2006). The MMPI was introduced in 1943 and was the sole MMPI instrument for 46 years until the MMPI-2 was published in 1989 (Butcher et al., 1989, 2001). The MMPI's normative sample included only White people. Using this racially biased instrument to assess and draw conclusions about Black people and other People of Color deprived them of a fair and unbiased assessment, whether in forensic, clinical, or other areas. One study of people living in a rural setting illustrates how profoundly distorted the results could be when an instrument normed on one group is used to assess a different group: All Black participants answered a particular MMPI item one way; all White participants answered the same item a different way. A widely used computerized service that scored and interpreted MMPI protocols processed the raw data in this study, falsely classifying 90% of the seemingly "normal" Black participants as psychiatric patients (Erdberg, 1970, 1988; Gynther et al., 1971). Thomas Faschinbauer (1979) summarized the issue bluntly:

> The median individual in that group had an eighth-grade education, was married, lived in a small town or on a farm, and was employed as a lower-level clerk or skilled tradesman. None was under 16 or over 65 years of age, and all were White. As a clinician I find it difficult to justify comparing anyone to such a dated group. When the person is 14 years old, Chicano, and lives in Houston's poor fifth ward, use of the original norms seems sinful. (p. 215; see also Pope et al., 2006)

This chapter discussed important areas to consider before entering the forensic work realm. The chapters that follow explore other important aspects of forensic work related to therapist–patient sexual involvement. The following questions may help us engage with the material we have just covered and see the implications for our work.

AN INVITATION FOR SELF-REFLECTION AND GROWTH

- What experience have you had with attorneys, courts, and the legal process? How do you think this might affect your work in this area?

- How familiar are you with the rules and procedures (e.g., rules of evidence) of the civil, administrative, and criminal courts in your jurisdiction? What steps, if any, will you take to learn this information and fill any gaps in knowledge?

- How do you select assessment instruments to ensure that they are not biased for the person you are assessing?

- What process could you create to identify and address your bias blind spots?
- What worries, fears, or concerns arise when considering the contrast between engaging in forensic versus clinical work with clients? How can we best navigate any emerging emotions and thoughts?
- Pause for a moment to reflect on your reactions to the topic of patient–therapist sexual involvement. Do you find yourself experiencing discomfort, anxiety, confusion, or other emotions? Are you troubled that these behaviors might be present among colleagues in our profession, possibly evoking a sense of guilt?
- How can you identify and address them to minimize the risk of impacting your forensic work?

RESOURCES

We have compiled diverse resources that readers may find helpful. They include the following:

- Specialty Guidelines for Forensic Psychology (American Psychological Association, 2013)
- Empirically Supported Forensic Assessment (Archer et al., 2016)
- Assessment of Test Bias on the MMPI-2-RF Higher Order and Restructured Clinical Scales as a Function of Gender and Race (Baker et al., 2023)
- Recommendations for the Use of Telepsychology in Psychology-Law Practice and Research: A Statement by American Psychology-Law Society (Batastini et al., 2023)
- Using the MMPI-3 in Legal Settings (Ben-Porath et al., 2022)
- *Testifying in Court: Guidelines and Maxims for the Expert Witness* (Brodsky, 2023)
- Feedback in Forensic Mental Health Assessment (Brodsky & Goldenson, 2022)
- Common Flaws in Forensic Reports (Brodsky & Pope, 2023)
- Adapting Assessment Processes to Consider Cultural Mistrust in Forensic Practices: An Example With the MMPI Instruments (Dixon et al., 2023)

- Trauma-Informed Forensic Mental Health Assessment: Practical Implications, Ethical Tensions, and Alignment With Therapeutic Jurisprudence Principles (Goldenson et al., 2022)

- The Practice of Clinical Forensic Psychology in Canada: Current Landscape and Future Directions (Goldenson et al., 2023)

- Computerized Test Interpretation of the MMPI-2 in the Forensic Context: A Time to Use Your Head and Not the Formula? (Lawson et al., 2022)

- Income, Demographics, and Life Experiences of Clinical-Forensic Psychologists in the United States (Neal & Line, 2022)

- Race-Informed Forensic Mental Health Assessment: A Principles-Based Analysis (Ratkalkar et al., 2023)

- Forensic Assessment Instruments: Their Reliability and Applicability to Criminal Forensic Issues (Rogers et al., 2023)

8

THE THERAPIST AS WITNESS

Indispensable First Steps When Working With Attorneys

The role of the expert witness carries profound responsibilities. If we fulfill these responsibilities, members of the jury may be able to understand complex concepts, complicated research studies, and unexpected patterns of behavior that are typically beyond the basic knowledge of the lay public. So much can depend on our testimony. Clear, informed, unbiased testimony can help someone whom a therapist has sexually exploited find some measure of justice in the legal system. It can help an accused therapist who has done nothing wrong clear their name and resume their career with the prospect of a trial and possible penalties no longer hanging over their head.

Sometimes, experts are appointed by the court, but more typically, they are hired by the prosecution, plaintiff, or defense attorneys. The questions we ask and the decisions we make during our initial contact with attorneys can be key to fulfilling our responsibilities. So much of what happens when we enter the world of depositions, courtroom testimony, forensic reports, and evidence is influenced by what we do or fail to do during the initial communications with an attorney. Some attorneys are exceptionally skilled. They care deeply about their clients. They work hard and are honest, ethical,

https://doi.org/10.1037/0000443-009
Therapists' Sexual Feelings and Fantasies: Research, Practice, Ethics, and Forensics,
by K. S. Pope, N. Y. Chavez-Dueñas, and H. Y. Adames

and effective. Working with them and seeing their work up close can feel like a privilege. They can inspire us to do our best work. But of course, not all attorneys are the ideal, and we need to be alert, aware, and well-prepared to deal with the ploys of those who aren't. We'll discuss some of these ploys in the following section. Following that, we explore the essential elements of a written policy for responding to attorneys. Creating such a policy can be indispensable, providing a framework to avoid potential blunders. The chapter closes with an opportunity for self-reflection.

ATTORNEYS' INITIAL PLOYS

Spoiler alert: Not all attorneys have the best intentions in mind. It will undoubtedly shatter some of our idealized vision of attorneys to learn that not all are scrupulously ethical, honest, and straightforward. (If this shocks you, feel free to take a break and some deep breaths to recover.) Awareness of some of the tricky ploys attorneys may put into play as soon as you pick up the phone can enable you to act quickly and decisively to head off trouble.

Blocking You From the Case

An attorney may call you and ask if they can have just a minute of your time to answer a quick question. Unfailingly polite, eager to please, and open to new business, you agree. They describe a quick scenario and ask if you think the therapist behaved unethically. You give a quick, top-of-the-head impression full of qualifications. A day or two later, you've forgotten about it. The attorney in this scenario had no interest in your answer and no interest in hiring you as an expert. Their call was part of a strategy to block you from being hired by the other side. Somewhere down the line, if you're named as an expert by the other side and are ready to testify on the basis of your extensive review of documents and forensic assessment of the other side's client, the attorney who originally called you will object to your testifying in light of your apparent conflict of interest. They will remind you (and the opposing attorney and court) that you had already consulted on the case for the attorney who called you. What may have seemed like just a few sentences of abstract description will be described as the very heart of their strategy and facts about the case you could not otherwise have learned. The attorney who called you will have contemporaneous documentation of the phone consultation, describing it in a way that makes it clear you cannot now testify for the other side.

Getting Your Consultation Without Paying

Like the attorney in the previous scenario, this attorney asks for just a minute of your time. But the "quick question" turns out to be somewhat complex, and the attorney fills in the background. Your response includes the necessary qualifications, conditionals, nuances, and reservations. Time passes. Imagine a movie scene in which the pages fly off the calendar on the wall. What seemed like a single question showing up at your office turns out, once it gets its foot in the door, to have brothers and sisters, aunts and uncles, distant cousins of all kinds forming a black hole in your day, sucking the time and energy you needed for other matters on your schedule. When you tell the attorney that you need to go, the attorney thanks you profusely for your time and then, like the television detective Columbo pausing on the way out, says, "Oh, and just one more thing."

Attorneys seeking free professional information and opinions draw on all sorts of strategies to obtain what is sometimes called "curbside consultations": flattery and other appeals to our ego, falsely implying that the conversation is our audition to be hired as an expert, playing on our impulse to be kind to someone who needs our help, and so on. However, jumping in and beginning to respond without taking the key steps outlined later in this chapter can open us up to a world of trouble.

Finding Out Confidential Information

An attorney—or someone working in an attorney's office—may call saying they just want to verify information that they already have. Their questions may include variations of the following:

- "[Name of a former client of yours] is suing their employer for discrimination. Am I right that you were their therapist?"

- "I just wanted to verify that you're [your first and last name], [your client's name]'s therapist—is that correct?"

- "Thanks for taking my call. I'm involved in a legal case regarding someone who was a patient of yours. I'm not asking you to reveal any confidential information, but I just wanted to check that they are no longer your patient—are they?"

Therapists should provide patients and former patients privacy, even regarding basic information such as whether the person is or was in therapy. This is even more important because the caller requesting the information may be an attorney representing someone who is suing the client, a private detective, or a reporter.

Sending You a Subpoena

Sometimes, attorneys will dispense with the personal introduction and simply subpoena the records of one of your clients or former clients. Therapists who have not had experience responding to subpoenas may be intimidated by the formal language of this legal document. It may make them anxious and eager to comply without delay. However, this impulse to reflexively comply opens the door to serious mistakes. Taking key steps before responding is crucial. In the following section, we provide information about how to respond to subpoenas.

THE WELL-PREPARED THERAPIST: PREPARATION AND RESPONSE

Having a clear policy for responding to attorneys is indispensable. If the policy is written and easily accessible whenever an attorney contacts you, it can help you stay organized and make sure you don't overlook anything important. Consider how you can adapt each of the following items into a written policy that fits you and your practice.

Documentation

Document every initial contact with an attorney, including the time and date of the contact and what was said. What may seem memorable during a call can fade in the weeks and months that follow, errors can creep in, facts can drop out, and material can get mixed up with other calls, cases, and consults. The ability to refresh (and correct) our memory later and, if needed, produce contemporaneous documentation can be crucial.

Who Is Calling and Why?

Attorneys are often skilled—or at least experienced—at persuasion and taking control of a discussion. If the attorney does not provide key information at the start of the phone call, the therapist must be ready before answering questions to ask the attorney to provide the following information:

- Who does the attorney represent?
- What case is this regarding?
- Why are they calling (e.g., for a consultation, to discuss hiring you as an expert)?
- How did they get your name?

Competence

If the attorney is calling to explore possibly hiring you as an expert witness, competence is a crucial consideration. An attorney may seek to hire you to testify as an expert witness on any of a diverse array of issues involving therapist–patient sexual involvement, including the following:

- Is a therapist who tells a client that they are the most attractive person the therapist has ever met (or that the client might feel better were they to loosen up and wear more revealing clothing or that the therapist believes therapeutic progress will begin once the client feels free to describe their sexual fantasies in detail) acting unethically, no matter what the circumstances or therapeutic orientation?

- Is a therapist who gives the client a hug and kiss at the beginning and end of every session behaving unethically, no matter the circumstances or therapeutic orientation?

- Is a therapist who asks a client who has had a sex change operation what it was like engaging in sex before and after the transition behaving unethically?

- Is a therapist who engages in sex with a client 1 month after termination behaving unethically no matter what the circumstances, theoretical orientation, or therapeutic method? How about 4 months? Six months? A year? Is there a time limit after which the behavior will no longer be considered unethical?

- Is a therapist who tells a client that they've had sexual fantasies about the client doing anything wrong?

- Is a therapist who has told a consultant that for months they've continued to have powerful, persistent sexual fantasies about a client and enjoyed those fantasies while masturbating but refused to consider the consultant's strong recommendation to transfer the client to another therapist violating the standard of care?

- Is a male therapist who has an obvious erection almost every session behaving unethically?

- Is a female therapist who wears an extremely low-cut blouse or high skirt acting unethically?

- Does a client who engages in sex with a therapist always suffer harm? Does sex with a therapist ever benefit the client?

- Can adult clients ever truly consent to sexual involvement with a current or former therapist?

Before agreeing to testify as an expert, we must ask ourselves if we possess genuine expertise in the relevant areas. What is our education, training, and supervised experience in each area? What work (e.g., research, publications, teaching) have we done in the areas? Have we stayed up to date on the theory and research and the ethical, professional, and legal standards in these areas?

Authorization to Release Information

If the attorney calls you out of the blue, claims they represent one of your current or former clients, and begins to ask you questions about the therapy or client, politely explain that your policy is not to provide information—even about whether someone is a current or former client—unless you have a signed and dated release of information form. Request that they fax or otherwise deliver the form to you so that you can verify it before responding.

If you receive the form, contact the former or current client before responding to the attorney. Ensure the documented consent is truly informed and current (e.g., have they subsequently revoked their consent?). Does the client understand the implications of your submitting their therapy notes to a third party or testifying in a public proceeding about them and their case?

Subpoena

Therapists may receive a subpoena to produce documents such as billing and treatment records. This is known as a *subpoena duces tecum*. Or they may be subpoenaed to testify in a deposition, trial, or other procedure. This is known as a *subpoena ad testificandum*.

Adames, Chavez-Dueñas, Vasquez, and Pope (2023) identified three fundamental mistakes therapists can make when they receive a subpoena:

- They toss it into the stack of "these are not due right this second, so I'll get around to them when I have a little extra free time." Readers are invited to speculate on how long it takes a therapist these days before they experience "a little extra free time"—if they ever do.

- They feel anxious or intimidated by the legal language or just want to get this matter off their to-do list as soon as possible and quickly send off the requested documents before

  - reading the subpoena carefully,
  - consulting with their attorney, and
  - considering if there are legitimate reasons not to comply.

- They forget to inform the client or former client early so that the client understands what is happening, can object to releasing information about them, and, if necessary, hire an attorney to attempt to quash or limit the subpoena.

Therapists should never simply assume that because of certain circumstances, a client need not be informed that their records have been subpoenaed. In one case, a woman filed a licensing complaint against her therapist, who then subpoenaed her records from her present and former physicians, therapists, and even former attorneys without prior notice to the woman. When the woman discovered that her records had been disclosed, she took the matter to court. According to the court's published opinion, the woman:

> complained to the Board of Psychology of the State of California about . . . a licensed clinical psychologist. The Board initiated disciplinary action against [the psychologist] and a hearing was set before an administrative law judge. . . . In anticipation of the hearing, [the psychologist] served 17 or more subpoenas duces tecum on [the woman's] past and present physicians and psychotherapists and her former attorneys. Copies of the subpoenas were served on the Board, but no notice of any kind was given to [the woman]. The records were produced to the ALJ [Administrative Law Judge] at a preheating conference and the ALJ gave them to [the psychologist's] attorney.
>
> When [the woman] discovered the disclosure, she filed a petition for a writ of mandate to compel the Department of General Services to quash the subpoenas and return the documents. The Board of Psychology (as one real party in interest) did not oppose the petition and disclaimed any interest in [the woman's] personal records. [The psychologist] (the other real party in interest) claimed the petition was moot because the disciplinary action had been settled but nevertheless insisted the records had been properly subpoenaed. . . .
>
> The trial court granted the petition, finding service of the subpoenas without prior notice to [the woman] violated her rights of privacy, and ordered [the psychologist] to pay [the woman's] attorneys' fees of $70,830. (*Sehlmeyer v. Department of General Services*, 1993, p. 1075)

The psychologist had put forth various complex arguments based on what was and was not included in state laws and regulations. The appellate court noted that they had not attempted to resolve all the issues because, even if the psychologist was correct, "there still exists a constitutional and common law right to privacy, which resolves the underlying issue against [the psychologist]" (*Sehlmeyer v. Department of General Services*, 1993, p. 1077).

It is important to note that the courts have not always treated this right to privacy as absolute. In one case of an alleged romantic relationship between a therapist and his former patient, the court held that the state had a compelling interest that outweighed the former patient's right to privacy:

> After receiving formal written complaints that the psychiatrist and his former patient were having a romantic relationship, and the psychiatrist was depressed and abusing alcohol, State Board of Physical Quality Assurance initiated investigation and subpoenaed psychiatrist's records relating to patient's treatment. Psychiatrist filed motion to quash subpoena [which was denied]. Patient filed motion for reconsideration which was denied. . . . The Court of Special Appeals . . . held that: (1) Board had authority to begin investigation on basis of complaints, notwithstanding contention that matter was beyond the scope of Board's authority because personal relationship between psychiatrist and patient began after doctor-patient relationship terminated; (2) fact that patient had not complained about psychiatrist's behavior did not preclude disciplinary investigation; and (3) patient could not assert her constitutional right to privacy to bar disclosure to Board of records of her treatment by psychiatrist, as right to privacy was outweighed by state's compelling interest. (*Dr. K v. State Board of Physician Quality Assurance*, 1993, p. 453)

To summarize, we provide seven important actions to consider when responding to a subpoena, including the following:

- Deal with it promptly. Don't set it aside, delay responding to it, or forget about it.

- Don't impulsively, reflexively, and immediately send off the records without first taking the other steps listed here.

- Read the subpoena carefully, and make sure you understand what it is asking for.

- Consider whether there are legitimate reasons not to comply.

- Consult your attorney.

- Notify your client or former client.

- Consult the "Strategies for Private Practitioners Coping With Subpoenas or Compelled Testimony for Client/Patient Records or Test Data or Test Materials" Committee on Legal Issues, American Psychological Association (2016), which is included in this book as Resource G.

Conflicting Roles

Remaining alert to actual and apparent conflicts of roles is an essential ethical and professional responsibility. One of the most common dilemmas confronting therapists is when a lawyer representing one of the therapist's clients or former clients tries to get the therapist to testify as both a fact witness and an expert witness. These two distinct roles conflict:

> Attempting to treat and evaluate the same person typically creates a role conflict. This role conflict manifests itself in different conceptions of truth and causation, different forms of alliance, different types of assessment, and different ethical guidelines. Although circumstances sometimes compel a practitioner to assume the dual role of treater and evaluator, the problems that surround this practice argue for its avoidance whenever possible. (Strasburger et al., 1997, p. 448; see also Gutheil & Brodsky, 2008)

Both beginning and experienced witnesses may feel that they are competent to bridge the conflicts and avoid the resulting bias by remaining alert and conscientious. However, as Greenberg and Shuman (2007) observed,

> To perform a competent forensic examination, the expert must not only possess the requisite skills and expertise to perform the tasks of the examination, the expert must also exercise the untainted and unbiased judgment that is likely to become impaired when one provides both therapeutic and forensic services to the same individual. As to the argument that such taint and bias inherent in such dual roles can be avoided by expertise and mental resolve, one need only to be familiar with writings such as Fischhoff (1982), Koriat, Lichtenstein, and Fischhoff (1980), Slovic and Fischhoff (1977), and Gilovich, Griffin, and Kahneman (2002) to appreciate that one's attempts to argue with oneself against being biased are not adequate antidotes to that bias. (p. 131)

Gutheil and Drogin (2013) summed up the major issues succinctly by describing how "in general, these two roles—treater and expert—are considered incompatible because the clinical, legal, and ethical mandates are markedly different for each" (p. 3).

Payment

Each of us has financial needs, responsibilities, wants, and limitations. Our styles in setting and collecting fees differ from each other. It is important to have a clear fee policy and negotiate the amount, method, and expected time of payments for work as an expert witness before the work begins. For example, both parties should explicitly agree, preferably in writing, on such issues as the following:

- Will the expert be paid by the hour or a lump sum for specific tasks, such as conducting a forensic psychological assessment and submitting a report?

- Will the expert be paid any or all of the fee in advance or only after the work is completed?

- Who is responsible for paying the expert, making sure the payment is on time, and so on?

- It is worth noting that the fees for fact witnesses and the payment method are usually set by laws or formal procedures in the relevant jurisdiction.

AN INVITATION FOR SELF-REFLECTION AND GROWTH

- Before reading this chapter, how did you envision managing subpoenas, or have you had any experience handling them? What influenced your response?

- Imagine you are a therapist creating a comprehensive written policy for responding to subpoenas. What steps would you include in your policy?

- Have you encountered any tricky ploys from attorneys in the past? If you have, would your response differ after reading the insights from this chapter? What actions would you maintain, and what alterations would you make?

- Imagine you are a therapist creating a comprehensive written policy for responding to phone calls from attorneys asking you for information about a current or former client or seeking to hire you as a fact or expert witness. What steps would you include in the policy?

- Imagine you are a forensic practitioner in solo practice, creating a written policy for responding to initial phone calls from attorneys. What steps would your policy include?

- Take a moment to reflect on how it benefits you, your practice, and your clients to be prepared when working with attorneys.

9 FORENSIC PSYCHOLOGICAL ASSESSMENT AND REPORT

Serving as an expert witness is a complex role with many moving parts. It involves conducting forensic evaluations that draw on multiple sources of information, including a comprehensive record review, interviews to obtain collateral information, empirically validated psychological testing, and measures of the client's effort or motivation during testing. The evaluator then prepares a written report integrating the findings to answer the psycho–legal referral question.

This chapter outlines important considerations to keep in mind when performing an evaluation and writing a report as an expert witness in cases involving therapist–patient sexual involvement.

AN EXPLICIT SHARED PURPOSE

A competent forensic psychological assessment begins with a clear understanding of the evaluation's purpose. This essential first step can be easily overlooked in the quick abstractions and generalities batted back and forth

https://doi.org/10.1037/0000443-010
Therapists' Sexual Feelings and Fantasies: Research, Practice, Ethics, and Forensics,
by K. S. Pope, N. Y. Chavez-Dueñas, and H. Y. Adames

between attorney and clinician, each assuming the other mirrors their understanding. It is critical to make the goal of the evaluation explicit to prevent any confusion or potential misunderstandings. Consider the following questions:

- Why is the attorney asking for an assessment?
- What, exactly, do they want to find out?
- What questions do they want answered or at least addressed?

If a psychological assessment is unlikely to answer—or cannot answer—one or more of those questions, make sure the attorney knows this before the evaluation begins. Many attorneys multitask and may not devote all their attention to a discussion. Documenting the purpose in writing is an additional layer of assurance, ensuring both parties are aligned. Providing a written record allows each of you to review and confirm that it covers everything the attorney believes is important. This document can prevent later disputes caused by the frailties of memory. It can head off "But I asked you to assess something different from what is in your report," or "As I remember, you asked me to assess x, y, and z, not a, b, and c."

SETTING FEES

Once you've agreed to conduct a psychological assessment, the next step involves establishing your fees. If you and the hiring attorney have not yet reviewed and signed a separate document outlining the fees, their calculation method (e.g., whether you charge by the hour, by the report, or in some other way), payment details, and so forth, consider incorporating these specifics into a document as part of the purpose of the assessment.

A common misstep is underestimating how long it will take to prepare, review, and submit the report. Kahneman (2011) wrote,

> Overly optimistic forecasts of the outcome of projects are found everywhere. Amos and I coined the term *planning fallacy* to describe plans and forecasts that are unrealistically close to best-case scenarios. . . . Examples of the planning fallacy abound in the experiences of individuals, governments, and businesses. The list of horror stories is endless. (p. 249)

Hitches are not uncommon in forensic assessments: A client fails to show up for an assessment session (or shows up so late you can get little done); you have car trouble, get sick, or have an emergency at home and miss an assessment session; your computer (which you need to score the raw data and to write and print your report) crashes or there is a Wi-Fi outage; the assessment turns out to be more complicated than you'd imagined and you need to administer, score, and interpret additional tests; you have trouble tracking down and obtaining the prior records to review, and on and on and on. When estimating the time you will need to prepare a report, be sure to factor in time for the surprises you'll likely encounter.

PRIOR RECORDS

Although the need to review particular records or interview third parties may not emerge until the assessment is underway, the clinician should try to anticipate the need for time in this area. For example, in the case of someone who alleges sexual contact with a prior therapist and alleges that the contact resulted in psychological harm, previous records of psychological evaluations, diagnosis, and treatment may be critical elements of the assessment. Preliminary discussions with the attorney should specify whether the attorney or clinician will be responsible for gathering the necessary records, as well as a reasonable timeline for getting them.

UNANTICIPATED REVELATIONS INVOLVING MANDATED REPORTING

Each state and province has its own set of legislation and case law governing mandated reporting in such areas as child abuse and threats to third parties. Part of professional competence is being aware of these professional duties. A forensic assessment may turn up information requiring the clinician to notify law enforcement, the Department of Child Welfare Services, or other appropriate agencies within a short time frame. This legal mandate may put the clinician in conflict with the attorney who retained them to conduct the evaluation. The attorney may direct the clinician not to disclose the information to the appropriate agency or any third parties because the information is a work product or information collected and prepared to be used in a legal matter, which is often protected by the attorney–client privilege. In these instances, the attorney may argue that privilege takes precedence. It is best to address these potential conflicts before the evaluation begins. The clinician and attorney need to agree on the clinician's responsibilities if the assessment turns up information meeting the criteria for mandated reporting. The agreement should be in writing to prevent misunderstandings. If the clinician and attorney cannot agree, it may be best for the clinician to decline to conduct the assessment.

ASSESSMENT INSTRUMENT NORMS, VALIDITY, AND RELIABILITY

Once clear arrangements have been made with the attorney, we begin selecting the assessment instruments and approaches that make the most sense—in light of the research data and our professional opinion—for assessing this particular individual and answering the referral question(s). Check the norming, validity, and reliability of each instrument for this person. Does the research demonstrate that the instrument performs well with people who match this person's

- gender,
- age group,
- language skills,
- reading ability,
- special circumstances (e.g., blind, deaf, mobility impaired),
- racial group, and
- culture(s)?

If you encounter a situation where you can't identify and obtain instruments that are valid and reliable for assessing a client, there are several actions you can consider, including the following:

- Consult with colleagues with expertise in conducting psychological assessments with people from the client's cultural and linguistic background.

- Look for any available normative data in the language the client speaks and the country the client comes from, preferably with adjusted norms for gender, age, and education.

- Identify and use measures free from cultural and linguistic biases (e.g., Test of Nonverbal Intelligence, Color Trails Test).

- Ensure your report clearly communicates your actions and describes how tests lacking specific normative data for the client likely underrepresent their performance and abilities.

- Consider the cultural and racialized equivalence of psychological measures when interpreting psychological data and reaching conclusions (Helms, 1992, 2015; see also Adames, Chavez-Dueñas, & Jernigan, 2023).

INFORMED CONSENT

The formal assessment process begins once informed consent has been obtained. A simple way to start this process is to ask the patient if they understand why they're meeting with you. Some may have been told by the attorney's secretary that the attorney wants them to contact you for an appointment, often with limited details. Consequently, patients might feel uncertain about the reason for meeting with you. For this reason, it is important that you allow time to explain to patients the purpose of the evaluation, providing them with information about who you are, what you do, and what is involved in the psychological evaluation. If you are writing a report and testifying, describe who will have access to the report and ask if they have any concerns about that. It is crucial that they understand the degree to which everything they say is—or is not—subject to confidentiality and privilege and what the exceptions are.

Videoconferencing

The informed consent should cover the use of videoconferencing technology if the assessment sessions will not be in person. Planning this aspect of the consent process provides an excellent opportunity for the clinician to review their competence in using Zoom or other software to conduct an assessment and their awareness of the current literature in this area (e.g., Abascal et al., 2023; Batastini et al., 2023; Goldenson & Josefowitz, 2021; Palfreman, 2023).

Recordings and Third-Party Observers

The informed consent should also address whether the assessment will be recorded (audio, video, or both) or observed by one or more third parties. Adequately informing the person to be assessed requires each of us to be informed about the evolving policies, position statements, and other literature in this area (e.g., Boone et al., 2022; Glen et al., 2021; Lewandowski et al., 2016; Siegel & Kinscherff, 2018). A particularly useful article is "Third Party Observers: The Effect Size Is Greater Than You Might Think" (Gavett et al., 2005; see also Howe & McCaffrey, 2010; Rezaei et al., 2017; Yantz & McCaffrey, 2009).

ADEQUATE AND ACCURATE NOTES

Professionals conducting forensic assessments are responsible for preserving adequate information. The opposing attorney will carefully examine notes and other records of the assessment, looking for gaps, mistakes, and misleading statements—anything that might help them win the case by discrediting or casting doubt on the expert or the expert's report. The deposition and courtroom testimony may come years after you've conducted and written up your assessment. All the information and interactions may seem sharp and crisp in your mind in the immediate aftermath of the assessment. But later, these memories may have been tattered or devastated by the passage of time. In one instance, a psychologist appeared in court several years after the assessment. During cross-examination, they were asked to describe the client. The psychologist had comprehensive records of the test data and inferences based on those data but had never written anything about the patient's appearance. The psychologist had to admit that they didn't know if the client was about four feet or over six feet tall and could not remember if the person weighed under 120 or over 260 pounds (Pope et al., 2006).

THE REPORT

The forensic assessment report carries a heavy burden. An excellent report may bring justice to deserving people, helping them to recover and become whole. A flawed report may knock the quest for justice off course, adding injustice and hurt to people who have been harmed. It may allow those who caused that harm to get away with something and proclaim far and wide that they were innocent of doing anything wrong, they were the real victims, and they were wrongly the target of a witch hunt.

Forensic assessment reports should be comprehensive, specific, and transparent. They should clearly describe every step in the process and provide a firm basis for the conclusions.

Good reports are organized and written in a manner that's easy to understand. Professional jargon can often confuse rather than clarify, especially when the reader is an attorney, judge, or juror who is completely unfamiliar with those terms. Try to use everyday language. It is important to honestly disclose any factors that may threaten the validity of the evaluation. Data that do not neatly fit the conclusions should be acknowledged and discussed.

For those who would like more detailed guidance on writing forensic reports, please see S. Brown et al. (2017), DeMier and Otto (2017), Karson and Nadkarni (2013), Otto et al. (2014), Pope et al. (2006), and Zwartz (2018).

In closing this section, we leave you with Brodsky and Pope's (2023) seven principles for writing better forensic assessment reports and avoiding common pitfalls:

1. Humility is essential. Many flawed reports are caused by excessive pride and a lack of humility. All of us are presumably proud of our hard-won skills and experience, and good reports reveal appropriate confidence. After all, if we do not view ourselves as experts, it may be difficult for the court to view us as experts and admit us to testify as expert witnesses. Nevertheless, humility includes reminding ourselves that we all have weaknesses as well as strengths and that it is hard to be completely aware of our own biases and blind spots. That means taking the time to review draft reports, making a fearless inventory of the flaws, questionable assertions, and areas for improvement.

2. For all tests, scales, and so forth, double-check the math, scoring, and so forth. It can be agonizing to watch a colleague—or to be that expert—squirm in the witness chair as a brutal cross-examination highlights an error in calculating an intelligence scale score or translating a score into the wrong category, undermining the report's conclusions and the court's confidence in the expert. Perhaps it is worse when such errors go undetected, sometimes affecting lives and possibly just verdicts.

3. Check to make sure all significant conditions of the assessment and their effects on the assessment are clearly identified and discussed. Examples are if the assessment was in English, which is the examinee's newly acquired second language; the session was audiotaped or video-taped; third parties were looking or listening in; or loud construction or personnel sounds intruded.

4. Place yourself in the shoes of each person whose life may be affected by your report. If you were those people, would you believe that the assessment was conducted and reported fairly and appropriately? How would you criticize the report from their point of view—are any of those criticisms valid?

5. Try to poke holes in the draft report's clarity, completeness, and conclusions. Is it clear how the assessment was conducted, who conducted the assessment, what versions of what instruments were used, and how you arrived at the results (e.g., relying on computerized scoring and interpretation, using algorithms)? Check whether your conclusions rest firmly on the data and whether you have properly qualified your conclusions.

6. Seek out directed feedback. Few forensic mental health professionals get pointed, specific, and critical feedback on their reports. Why? Because most write reports alone, without collaboration. Because most cases are settled or plea-bargained and challenges in the form of truly tough and knowledgeable cross-examinations are rare. Because even when the cross-examinations are tough, few go after how the report is written, and few experts actually go back and rethink how they write.

7. Provide and receive consultation. When we searched the literature for forensic psychology consultation and forensic psychiatry consultation, we found many articles about psychologists offering consultation to attorneys, to the court, and to agencies. We found nothing on consultation with other forensic mental health professionals on report writing. We have offered occasional consultation to testifying experts but have never been sought out

about the immediate quality of the reports. The consultation always began with others reaching out for assistance in preparing for court testimony. Then the nature of the report is brought up as preparation for testimony. Intense discussion often follows about how the evaluation is conducted and how the report is written. The bottom-line suggestion is that assessors reexamine the organization, structure, presentation of data, conclusions, opinions, and length of reports. Forensic examiners can change how they write reports. But it almost always calls for some external or forceful event. (p. 416)

AN INVITATION FOR SELF-REFLECTION AND GROWTH

- What are your thoughts and reactions about the process of conducting psychological assessments with patients alleging sexual involvement with therapists?

- How does the experience of being an expert witness differ when working within the realm of therapist–patient sexual involvement compared with other areas you've previously practiced in?

- What additional data might you consider adding to your psychological reports that perhaps you did not include in the past?

- After engaging with the material in this chapter, are there any adjustments you would consider making in your approach to conducting assessments and writing reports?

10 TESTIFYING EFFECTIVELY

Navigating Humility, Responsibility, and Both Cognitive and Emotional Bias

Navigating the legal system can be stressful for many of us therapists. We go from the familiarity of our offices to the adversarial conflicts of the courtroom, where one of the attorneys will likely do their best to point out flaws in our work and discount or discredit our conclusions. Cases involving allegations of therapist–patient sex can bring an additional layer of discomfort. The tendency of this topic to throw us off balance, distorting our ability to think clearly and act responsibly, can gain force when we step out of the familiar world of the therapy office and enter the forensic realm with its different customs, rules, expectations, and objectives. The topic of the therapist's sexual feelings and behavior with clients has also, as previously documented, been one that the profession sometimes avoided or pushed out of sight, suppressing research results and protecting the reputation and welfare of the profession at the expense of the safety and well-being of clients.

This chapter offers information and suggestions to help therapists testify about therapist–patient sexual involvement confidently and effectively while managing their reactions and maintaining the highest professional and ethical standards.

https://doi.org/10.1037/0000443-011
Therapists' Sexual Feelings and Fantasies: Research, Practice, Ethics, and Forensics,
by K. S. Pope, N. Y. Chavez-Dueñas, and H. Y. Adames

ACTIVE HUMILITY

The research and history presented in this book describe an area loaded with snares, snags, and pitfalls for professionals. Early chapters emphasized that simply experiencing sexual attraction to a client can evoke anxiety, guilt, and confusion in many therapists. Later chapters showed that even famous and influential therapists have sometimes chosen to place their clients at risk of harm, violate ethics and the law, and risk their professional license and livelihood by starting a sexual relationship with a client. While we prepare to testify and during the actual proceedings, it is crucial to remain aware of these snares, snags, and pitfalls and keep in mind that we, too, are vulnerable to them.

Practicing active humility can prevent countless errors. It can be easy to assume that because we are familiar with this area, have extensive clinical or forensic experience, or feel confident, the snares, snags, and pitfalls present no threat to us personally. Active humility involves continuously reminding ourselves of our fallibility and vulnerabilities. It means constantly asking ourselves what other ways there are to view or understand the situation. What information might I be lacking, overlooking, or misreading? What mistakes could I be making? What steps could I take to be sure I'm on solid ground—or to learn that my conclusions are shaky? When we are unwilling to maintain humility and not be alert and vigilant, we place ourselves at the greatest risk of making blunders.

THE BASIC RESPONSIBILITY

Keeping in mind our basic responsibility as we step into the forensic realm is crucial. If we testify as a fact witness, we are there to report as clearly, accurately, and objectively as possible, in response to questions from the attorneys (and occasionally from the judge) what we saw, heard, or otherwise know about the events or facts relevant to the case. If we testify as expert witnesses, we are there to express, objectively and without bias, our professional opinions and conclusions. As experts, we help the trier of fact (usually the jury and sometimes the judge) understand highly complex clinical, technical, or scientific issues beyond the layperson's understanding.

Humility can help us stick with our basic responsibility during *deposition* (providing testimony under oath before the trial), *direct examination* (responding to questions from the attorney who asked the witness to testify), and *cross-examination* (responding to questions by the opposing party) and prevent us from using our testimony to try to

- become the star witness and center of attention;
- show off our intelligence, knowledge, authority, or verbal fluency;
- entertain the courtroom with our wit and engaging personality;
- impress everyone with how important we are;
- act as if we are an infallible know-it-all;
- outduel and shut down the attorney who cross-examines us;
- discredit the other experts who testified through scorn, ridicule, and personal insults; and
- achieve a predetermined desired outcome (e.g., supporting a colleague or patient to get justice).

THE BIAS BLIND SPOT IN FORENSIC TESTIMONY

Perhaps the greatest threat to our basic responsibility to testify objectively and without bias is the dreaded *bias blind spot* to which we are all vulnerable. In a foundational set of studies published over 2 decades ago, Emily Pronin and her colleagues demonstrated that

> knowledge of particular biases in human judgment and inference, and the ability to recognize the impact of those biases on others, neither prevents one from succumbing nor makes one aware of having done so. Indeed, our research participants denied that their assessments of their personal qualities (Study 2) and their attributions for a particular success or failure (Study 3) had been biased *even after having displayed the relevant biases and reading descriptions of them* [emphasis added]. (Pronin et al., 2002, p. 378)

Since then, many studies have explored, validated, and extended the sad truth that even learning about specific biases and believing that those biases can affect others does not necessarily prevent us from displaying those biases or make us aware that we've shown bias (e.g., Chandrashekar et al., 2021; Ehrlinger et al., 2005; Pronin & Hazel, 2023; Scopelliti et al., 2015; West et al., 2012; Zaleskiewicz & Gasiorowska, 2021).

Studies have shown the bias blind spot at work in the forensic area. For example, Neal and Brodsky (2016) conducted a qualitative study with 20 board-certified forensic psychologists, followed by a survey of 351 forensic psychologists. They found that "evaluators perceived themselves as less vulnerable to bias than their colleagues, consistent with the phenomenon called the 'bias blind spot'" (p. 58). Kukucka et al. (2017) surveyed hundreds of experienced forensic examiners from 21 countries and found that

> overall, examiners regarded their judgments as nearly infallible and showed only a limited understanding and appreciation of cognitive bias. . . . Many examiners showed a *bias blind spot* . . . acknowledging bias in other domains but not their own, and in other examiners but not themselves. (p. 452)

Similarly, Zapf and colleagues (2018), in a survey of 1,099 mental health professionals who conduct forensic assessments for courts or other tribunals, found evidence for a bias blind spot, with more forensic mental health professionals seeing bias in their colleagues' judgments than their own. They also found that

> evaluators who had received training about bias were more likely to acknowledge cognitive bias as a cause for concern, whereas evaluators with more experience were less likely to acknowledge cognitive bias as a cause for concern in forensic evaluation as well as in their own judgments. (p. 1)

We may be even more likely to fall victim to a bias blind spot when we feel especially confident in our professional judgments or when we are among experts who have reached a consensus opinion. However, both confidence and consensus can be mistaken for signs of accuracy or validity (Dror et al., 2018).

Active humility is key in remaining aware that we are all vulnerable to bias blind spots no matter how vast our knowledge, experience, prestige, or self-admiration may be. The more confident we are in our work, the more it is worth asking ourselves if we are missing something. Any of us can find ourselves infected with what we'll call a *meta-blind spot*: We remain blissfully (and arrogantly) unaware that we could ever have bias blind spots.

EMOTIONAL BIAS AND BLIND SPOTS

It is often difficult for forensic professionals to become fully aware of their emotional reactions to the litigants and the themes of the litigation and how these reactions can lead to significant bias (e.g., Barros et al., 2014; Goldenson & Gutheil, 2023; Goldyne, 2007; Reeder & Schatte, 2011; Sattar et al., 2002; Schetky & Colbach, 1982). The adversarial setting—pitting the plaintiff against the defendant and the prosecution against the defense, with large amounts of money or freedom on the line—can assault the witness's emotional composure.

A classic textbook on cross-examination—still in use and in print through 12 editions more than a century after its original publication—uses humor and exaggeration to identify some of the pressures that push and pull on those who testify as expert or fact witnesses:

> Of all unfortunate people in this world, none are more entitled to sympathy and commiseration than those whom circumstances oblige to appear upon the witness stand in court. . . . You are [between two lawyers,] one of whom smiles at you blandly because you are on his side, the other eying you savagely for

the opposite reason. The gentleman who smiles, proceeds to pump you of all you know; and having squeezed all he wants out of you, hands you over to the other, who proceeds to show you that you are entirely mistaken in all your supposition; that you never saw anything you have sworn to . . . in short, that you have committed direct perjury. He wants to know if you have ever been in state prison, and takes your denial with the air of a man who thinks you ought to have been there, asking all the questions over again in different ways; and tells you with an awe-inspiring severity, to be very careful what you say. He wants to know if he understood you to say so and so, and also wants to know whether you meant something else. Having bullied and scared you out of your wits, and convicted you in the eye of the jury of prevarication, he lets you go. (Wellman, 1911, pp. 168–169)

Skilled attorneys can pick up on the slightest "tell" in the witness's behavior, voice patterns, verbal patterns, and demeanor, zeroing in on ambiguities, mistakes, and areas of discomfort. They exploit our emotional reactions to the stresses of testifying. One attorney described the signs that told "the cross-examiner to uncoil and strike" by stating the following:

Have you ever seen a "treed" witness? Have you ever had the experience of watching a witness's posterior involuntarily twitch? Have you ever seen them wiggle in their chairs? Have you ever seen their mouths go dry? Have you seen the beads of perspiration form on their foreheads? Have you ever been close enough to watch their ancestral eyes dilating the pupil so that they would have adequate tunnel vision of the target that was attacking? (Burgess, 1984, p. 252)

When encountering the snares, snags, and pitfalls that characterize the focus of this book, there are two major forms of emotional bias blind spots that clinicians entering the forensic arena can fall prey to: (a) a lack of adequate awareness of emotional reactions and (b) limited awareness of how emotional reactions create bias.

Lack of Adequate Awareness of Emotional Reactions

Earlier chapters in the book helped us reflect on the reactions of clinicians, the inappropriate behaviors of reputable therapists, and the silence of the professional community regarding the issue of sexual involvement between therapists and patients. We discussed how

- simply experiencing sexual attraction to a client can evoke feelings of anxiety, guilt, and confusion in many therapists, so we avoid thinking or talking about it;

- even famous and influential therapists have sometimes abused their power and chosen to place their clients at risk for harm, violated ethics and the law, and risked their license and livelihood by starting a sexual relationship with a client; and

- the profession sometimes avoided or silenced the topics covered in this book, suppressing research results and protecting the reputation and welfare of the discipline at the expense of the safety and well-being of clients.

Each of these three points suggests the kinds of emotional reactions that could potentially introduce bias into our forensic work. Imagine the following scenarios as vividly as possible and ask yourself what emotions you're experiencing. Try not to limit yourself to one emotion. Many of us experience a variety of emotional reactions to such situations, some of which bubble to the surface more slowly than others, some of which may be contradictory, and some which make us uncomfortable and eager to move on before they reach full awareness.

Scenario 1

You have been hired by an attorney representing a woman who entered therapy to deal with incest issues that had plagued her life. She reports that she was seduced by her therapist, which led to her divorce, loss of custody of her children, and a suicide attempt that resulted in hospitalization. As a result of your assessment, you believe her. Consider the following questions:

- What emotions are you aware of when you imagine this scenario?
- How might those emotions have led or contributed to bias in your assessment?
- How might each of those emotions create bias in your subsequent testimony?

Scenario 2

You have been hired by an attorney representing a woman who entered therapy to deal with incest issues that had plagued her life. She reports that she was seduced by her therapist, which led to her divorce, loss of custody of her children, and a suicide attempt that resulted in hospitalization. As a result of your assessment, you believe that there was no sexual activity between therapist and patient and that the patient's account of what she described as "seduction" was a psychotic delusion.

- What emotions are you aware of when you imagine this scenario?
- How might those emotions have led or contributed to bias in your assessment?
- How might each of those emotions create bias in your subsequent testimony?

Scenario 3

You have been hired by an attorney representing a woman who entered therapy to deal with incest issues that had plagued her life. She reports that she was seduced by her therapist, which led to her divorce, loss of custody of her children, and a suicide attempt that resulted in hospitalization. As a result of your assessment, you believe that there was no sexual activity between therapist and patient and that the patient's account is an elaborate lie to get money.

- What emotions are you aware of when you imagine this scenario?
- How might those emotions have led or contributed to bias in your assessment?
- How might each of those emotions create bias in your subsequent testimony?

Scenario 4

You have been hired by an attorney representing a therapist accused of engaging in sex with a client. This therapist is similar to you in many ways, and you find yourself identifying with the therapist.

- What emotions are you aware of when you imagine this scenario?
- How might those emotions have led or contributed to bias in your assessment?
- How might each of those emotions create bias in your subsequent testimony?

Scenario 5

You have been hired by an attorney representing a therapist accused of engaging in sex with a client. You find yourself sexually attracted to this therapist, experience persistent sexual fantasies about the therapist, and begin to imagine a relationship with the therapist once your participation in this legal matter has concluded.

- What emotions are you aware of when you imagine this scenario?
- How might those emotions have led or contributed to bias in your assessment?
- How might each of those emotions create bias in your subsequent testimony?

Scenario 6

You have been hired by an attorney representing a therapist accused of engaging in sex with a client. You find yourself sexually attracted to the client who is accusing the therapist and experience surprisingly arousing sexual fantasies about this client.

- What emotions are you aware of when you imagine this scenario?
- How might those emotions have led or contributed to bias in your assessment?
- How might each of those emotions create bias in your subsequent testimony?

Scenario 7

Are there any cultures, religious or spiritual beliefs, races, ethnicities, countries of origin, political views, socioeconomic backgrounds, class statuses, or characteristics you hold in high regard? If so, imagine you're presented with a case involving a party from such a background—how would you approach testifying in a case involving such a litigant?

- What emotions are you aware of when you imagine this scenario?
- How might those emotions have led or contributed to bias in your assessment?
- How might each of those emotions create bias in your subsequent testimony?

Scenario 8

Are there any cultures, religious or spiritual beliefs, races, ethnicities, countries of origin, political views, socioeconomic backgrounds, class statuses, or characteristics you hold negative feelings about? If so, imagine you are presented with a case involving a party from such a background—how would you approach testifying in a case involving such a litigant?

- If you had such negative feelings and imagined the case, what emotions are you aware of when you imagine this scenario?
- How might those emotions have led or contributed to bias in your assessment?
- How might each of those emotions create bias in your subsequent testimony?

Limited Awareness of How Emotional Reactions Create Bias

One of the most challenging bias blind spots—and one that gains strength from a lack of humility—is assuming that because we are aware of our emotional reactions, we can dismiss them as harmless to our objectivity and fairness. It is a human vulnerability to fail to see that we are not free from being biased by an emotional reaction. At the same time, it is pretty easy to notice how emotional responses can create bias in other people.

Consultation with a colleague who can view the matter objectively and be completely honest with us is often helpful, sometimes invaluable, in allowing us to avoid this trap. It may also be helpful to pay attention to our behavior (as opposed to our intentions) and see if we have been doing anything differently in this case.

COGNITIVE BIAS AND BLIND SPOTS

Adequate preparation for testimony involves reviewing the common sources of cognitive bias and identifying how they may have affected our work. This is important because if we are not careful about practicing humility, our testimony can go off track due to our cognitive bias and blind spots. The following are five of the most common sources of bias.

Adversarial Allegiance

Expert witnesses may sometimes be viewed as biased for the side that retained them (i.e., the attorney that is paying them). The most extreme version of this view is that they are "hired guns," ready to supply whatever testimony is wanted by the retaining attorney. But is this true? Does whichever side hired us matter if we're trying to be fair and objective in our testimony? Let's take a look at what research in this area says.

Murrie et al. (2013) paid 108 forensic psychologists and psychiatrists to examine the same offender case files. These forensic practitioners scored each offender on two widely used and extensively researched instruments that assessed risk. Half of the practitioners were told they were consulting for the defense; the other half were told they were working for the prosecution. Forensic psychologists and psychiatrists who believed they were working for the defense tended to assign lower risk scores to offenders than the forensic psychologists and psychiatrists who thought they were working for the prosecution, who tended to assign higher risk scores to those same offenders. This experiment and other investigations provide considerable evidence for an allegiance effect (McAuliff & Arter, 2016; Murrie et al., 2009; Murrie & Boccaccini, 2015; Otto, 1989; Perillo et al., 2021). Put simply, whichever side hired a practitioner seems to influence the conclusions the practitioner reaches.

Confirmation Bias

We return to Francis Bacon's iconic 1620 description of confirmation bias, cited previously in this book:

> The human understanding when it has once adopted an opinion . . . draws all things else to support and agree with it. And though there be a greater number and weight of instances to be found on the other side, yet these it either neglects or despises, or else by some distinction sets aside and rejects. (Bacon, 1955, p. 472)

When we assess one of the litigants, write our report, and prepare to testify, once we get a hypothesis we like, we are highly vulnerable to seeking, noticing, and emphasizing anything that supports that hypothesis and ignoring, discounting, or downplaying anything that disconfirms our hypothesis or suggests an alternative view.

Imagine that you have been hired as an expert witness on the case of a client who reported that their therapist coerced them into engaging in a sexual relationship with them. The client is a 19-year-old college student, and the therapist is a recently divorced 45-year-old man. The attorney asserts that the case is a "clear winner," considering the therapist abused his power to exploit the client for personal sexual gratification.

- What are your initial thoughts and reactions about the scenario?

- How might the information the attorney shared with you impact your evaluation, the questions you ask or don't ask, and the conclusions you reach?

- After reading the case, did you assume that the client is a woman? If so, why? If not, why not?

- Did you assume that the therapist was married to a woman? What influenced that assumption?

Hindsight Bias

Once we know how something turned out, we tend to imagine that we could have made a much better prediction about the result than had we tried to make the prediction beforehand (Arkes et al., 1988; Fischhoff, 1975; Fischhoff & Beyth, 1975; Guilbault et al., 2004; Salmen et al., 2023; Scurich et al., 2023; Wood, 1978). When evaluating the choices and other behaviors of any litigant, it can be challenging not to allow our knowledge of how the events turned out to improperly influence how we judge what they did. For example,

Janoff-Bulman et al. (1985) conducted experiments showing that hindsight bias can lead to blaming the victim.

Imagine you have been hired as an expert witness on the case of a client who reported that their therapist coerced them into engaging in a sexual relationship with them. The client is a 19-year-old college student, and the therapist is a recently divorced 45-year-old man. During your interview, the client shared that their experience began during the second therapy session when they started having flashbacks and sought comfort by asking their therapist for a hug.

- What reactions does this scenario evoke for you?
- What emotional reaction are you experiencing, and what thoughts come to mind when considering the client's request for a hug from their therapist?
- How are these reactions impacting your impressions of what happened and how this situation ended?
- How could an awareness of hindsight bias help in navigating situations resembling this scenario?

Narrative Bias

Narrative bias describes our tendency to create and believe narratives that explain why things happen by oversimplifying and overinterpreting. The concept of narrative bias

> addresses our limited ability to look at sequences of facts without weaving an explanation into them, or, equivalently, forcing a logical link, an *arrow of relationship*, upon them. Explanations bind facts together. They make them all the more easily remembered; they help them *make more sense*. Where this propensity can go wrong is when it increases our *impression* of understanding. (Taleb, 2010, p. 43; see also Taleb & Blyth, 2011)

Imagine that you have been hired as an expert witness on the case of a client who reported that their therapist coerced them into engaging in a sexual relationship with them. The client is a 19-year-old college student, and the therapist is a recently divorced 45-year-old man. After meeting with the client for the evaluation, you conclude that the therapist was likely seeking comfort from the client because they were going through a divorce. Later, it comes to light that this is not the therapist's first instance of allegedly engaging in sexual relationships with clients.

- What reactions does this scenario evoke for you?
- How did the narrative bias affect the conclusion reached by the therapist?
- What are some ways we can be vigilant in addressing narrative bias?

- What other factors could have influenced the therapist to violate the boundaries with the client?

What You See Is All There Is

Kahneman (2011) used WYSIATI to stand for "what you see is all there is." WYSIATI bias is our tendency to assume that what we currently know (or think we know) about something is all that exists. As expert witnesses, we rarely, if ever, have all the relevant information as the basis of our professional judgments and testimony. We must do our work without knowing all the facts and the whole story. We were not present during all the events at issue in the case. We must often rely on a patchwork of second-hand accounts (e.g., chart notes, interviews). We place ourselves at the highest risk for WYSIATI bias when we fail to ask ourselves what might be missing from our current knowledge, which would significantly change our understanding and professional opinions.

Imagine that you have been hired as an expert witness on the case of a client who reported that their therapist coerced them into engaging in a sexual relationship with them. The client is a 19-year-old college student, and the therapist is a recently divorced 45-year-old man. During your interview with the client, they presented as quiet, soft-spoken, and respectful. The client described the therapist as being cold, arrogant, and manipulative. As you review records, you come across a previous evaluation by a therapist describing the client as gregarious, talkative, and flirtatious.

- What are your initial thoughts and reactions about the scenario?

- How do you reconcile the difference between the client's behavior with you and their portrayal in the evaluation report by the previous therapist?

- How does this new information influence your perception of the client and their accusation regarding the alleged involvement of therapist–patient sexual involvement?

- What additional information may be useful in helping you better understand the case in this scenario?

Confidently and effectively testifying about therapist–patient sexual involvement, while upholding the highest professional and ethical standards, necessitates that we understand how we think, acknowledge, and manage emotional reactions and biases that can influence our work and cultivate active humility as a preventative measure against countless possible missteps.

MEETING THE CHALLENGES OF THE REAL WORLD

As this final part of the book draws to a close, an inescapable challenge comes into focus: How do we recognize and manage ethically and effectively the potential pitfalls of cognitive and emotional bias when we encounter them in the wild instead of the tame, captive pages of a book? We suggest you create your own personalized resource that includes the following:

- identifying what kinds of situations involving sexual feelings and fantasies might be most challenging for you to deal with ethically and effectively,

- identifying the kinds of cognitive and emotional bias that might be most challenging and potentially troublesome for you to recognize and manage,

- identifying the trusted professionals you would feel safe consulting when challenges seem daunting, and

- identifying your go-to rationalizations when you want to avoid recognizing your need for help coping with challenges.

We hope your journey through this book has been a helpful process of exploration, learning, and preparation. We hope it will help prepare you to meet the challenges of your clinical and forensic work in ways that meet the highest ethical, legal, and professional standards and, most important, your ideals.

PART **IV** INFORMED
CONSENT
RESOURCES

Resource A

INFORMED CONSENT FOR FORENSIC ASSESSMENT (WITH SPECIAL ATTENTION TO ISSUES OF THERAPIST–PATIENT SEXUAL INVOLVEMENT)[1]

The following document can be adapted to your practice, the specific legal case, and the client. Once you've adapted it, it's worth reviewing it to ensure it fits the client's ability to read and understand English. Specifically, ensure that the reading and comprehension levels of the document you've adapted match your client's reading proficiency in English. Finally, ask your attorney to read it to make sure it meets all the legal requirements in the jurisdiction where you practice.

*   *   *

Your attorney asked me to conduct a psychological assessment in connection with your court case, which involves issues related to sexual involvement with a previous therapist. This form was written to give you information about what will happen. The assessment will contain three main parts.

In the first part, which may take more than one session, I will give you several psychological tests. [Add a brief description of the tests.] We will

---

[1]This document has been adapted from *Sexual Involvement With Therapists: Patient Assessment, Subsequent Therapy, Forensics* (pp. 205–210), by K. S. Pope, 1994, American Psychological Association (https://doi.org/10.1037/10154-000). Copyright 1994 by the American Psychological Association.

discuss the instructions in detail before I give you the tests. It will be important that you understand the instructions for each test. If you don't understand the test's instructions, please let me know right away so I can better explain what the test is about.

In the second part, I will interview you. During the interview, I will ask you questions about yourself and ask you to talk about yourself. Some of the questions will be about what happened with your former therapist. There may, of course, be areas that you are reluctant to talk about. If there are any questions that you are uncomfortable answering or discussing during the interview, please be sure to let me know. Also, please let me know if you have any reasons for not providing the information. We can then talk about your concerns.

In the third part, I will describe my conclusions and review with you the information from the interview and tests you completed. You will have an opportunity to ask questions and discuss any opinions or information I review with you. During this time, I will invite you to comment on the information and my opinions. This will allow you to call my attention to anything you believe I got wrong and anything you think is incomplete or misleading. (It is possible, of course, that we may sometimes disagree.)

It is important that you be completely honest when responding to the items on the tests, providing information during the interview, and writing your response to the assessment. Information that is withheld, incomplete, wrong, or misleading may be more damaging than if I am able to get accurate information now and put it in context in my report or testimony. It is important for us to discuss any concerns you have in this area.

Although I will try to be thorough when I interview you, I may not ask about some areas or information that you believe are important. If so, please tell me so we can discuss them.

Please check each item below to indicate that you have read it carefully and understand it:

☐ I understand that Dr. _____ has been hired by my attorney, [fill in attorney's name], to conduct a psychological assessment for a case in which sexual involvement with a previous therapist is an issue.

☐ I understand that I will be asked to talk about the sexual involvement with a previous therapist, and I agree to do so.

☐ I understand that it is important for me to be honest and accurate when answering questions or providing information during this assessment.

☐ I understand that Dr. _____ may write a formal report about me based on the results of this assessment.

☐ I authorize Dr. _____ to send a copy of this formal report to my attorney and to discuss the report with them.

☐ I understand that Dr. _____ will not provide me with this written report but that I may, if I choose, schedule an additional appointment with Dr. _____ to discuss the results of this assessment.

☐ I authorize Dr. _____ to testify about me and this assessment in depositions and trial(s) related to my legal case.

☐ I understand that I may interrupt or discontinue this assessment at any time.

☐ I understand that even if I interrupt the assessment and it is not resumed or if I discontinue the assessment, it is possible (depending on the applicable laws, on rulings by the court, and/or on decisions by the attorneys in this case) that Dr. _____ may be called to submit a report or testify about the assessment, even if the assessment is incomplete.

☐ I understand that if I disclose certain types of special information to Dr. _____, they may be required or allowed to communicate this information to other people or agencies. As previously discussed with Dr. _____, examples of such information include reports of child or elder abuse and threats to kill or violently attack a specific person.

☐ I understand that the assessment will be audiotaped or videotaped.

☐ I understand that the audiotaped or videotaped record of the assessment will be given to my attorney and may become evidence in the deposition or trial(s).

If you have read, understood, and checked off each of the prior sections, please read carefully the following statement, and if you agree, please sign the statement. Do not sign if you have any questions that remain unanswered after we discuss them or if there are any aspects that you do not understand or agree to. Contact your attorney for guidance concerning how to proceed so that you fully understand the process and can decide whether you wish to continue.

Consent Agreement: I have read, agreed to, and checked off each of the previous sections. I have asked questions about any parts that I did not understand fully and any parts that I was concerned about. By signing below, I indicate that I understand and agree to the nature and purpose of this assessment, how it will be reported, and each of the points listed above.

Signature

_____

Name (please print)

_____

Date

_____

INFORMED CONSENT ISSUES FOR PROVIDING THERAPY TO PATIENTS WHO HAVE BEEN SEXUALLY INVOLVED WITH A PRIOR THERAPIST

As therapists, we hold informed consent as a vital ethical imperative. While informed consent may be thought of as something that is done at the beginning of therapy, we invite you to view it as a process rather than a static formality (Pope et al., 2021). The process is likely to occur differently and include different content depending on whether the therapy is, say, cognitive behavioral, psychodynamic, feminist, existential, systems, or gestalt. Aside from differences in theoretical orientation and technique, each therapist, patient, and situation is unique, requiring a personalized approach to informed consent that respects and accommodates these differences.

Although the process, both oral and written, will vary significantly from therapist to therapist, patient to patient, and setting to setting, certain issues seem central. What follows is a list of some of the most significant issues that tend to be part of the informed consent process. It may be helpful for the therapist to review this list periodically, considering the degree to which each issue may be essential to a particular patient in providing or withholding informed consent.

Because informed consent and therapy are processes, the list may be helpful not only at the beginning of therapy but also in subsequent stages as the patient's situation, therapeutic needs, and treatment plan change.

- Is there any evidence that the individual may not fully comprehend the information and issues relevant to giving or withholding informed consent?

- Are there any factors that would prevent this person from making decisions that are truly voluntary?

- Does the person adequately understand the type and nature of the services the therapist is offering?

- Are there alternative ways to effectively address the person's concerns, which could replace or supplement the therapy you provide? If so, is the person adequately aware of them?

- Suppose the degree of the therapist's education, training, or experience in providing clinical or forensic services to sexually exploited patients is relevant to the person's decision about whether to begin or continue work with the therapist. Does the person have the relevant information about the therapist?

- To the extent that the person has identified the previous therapist and other relevant individuals, groups, or organizations, has the new therapist ensured that there are no dual relationships, conflicts of interest, or role conflicts with the person's previous therapist or relevant individuals? Has the subsequent therapist disclosed any former or concurrent relationships that might affect the person's decisions about starting or continuing therapy with the new therapist?

- Does the person understand that the therapist is not an attorney and cannot provide legal counsel or representation?

- Does the person understand whether the therapist is licensed or, for instance, an unlicensed intern? Do they know the nature of the provider's license (e.g., psychology, psychiatry, or social work) and how the license status may affect issues such as types of services provided (e.g., medications), confidentiality, privilege, insurance coverage, and so forth?

- If any information about the person or the treatment will be communicated to or will be in any way accessible to others in your setting (e.g., administrative staff, utilization review committees, quality control personnel, or clinical supervisors) either orally (e.g., through supervision or case conferences) or in writing (e.g., through chart notes, treatment summaries, or treatment reports), is the person adequately aware of these communications and modes of access and their implications?

- If information about the person or treatment will be communicated to any payment source (e.g., an insurance company or a government agency), is the person adequately aware of the nature, content, and implications of these communications?

- Have any potential limitations in the number of sessions (e.g., a managed care plan's limit of 10 therapy sessions or an insurance plan's limitation of payments for mental health services to a specific dollar amount) or length of treatment (e.g., if the therapist is an intern whose internship will conclude within 3 months, after which the therapist will no longer be available) been adequately disclosed to the individual, and have the potential implications been adequately discussed?

- Does the person understand the therapist's policy regarding missed or canceled appointments?

- Has any information about the therapist that might significantly affect the person's decision to begin or continue work with the therapist been adequately disclosed and discussed? For example, a patient who has decided to start therapy and file a formal complaint to address sexual exploitation by a previous therapist may later feel betrayed if they learn only after a year of treatment and on the eve of trial (during which their subsequent therapist is expected to be a key witness) that the subsequent witness has frequently expressed the opinion that therapist–patient sexual involvement tends to benefit patients, has been sanctioned by an ethics committee, and has two licensing complaints pending.

- Does the person adequately understand limits to accessibility to the therapist (e.g., will the therapist be available to receive or return phone calls during the day, evenings, nights, weekends, or holidays)? Does the person adequately understand the limits of such accessibility between regularly scheduled sessions (e.g., will phone contacts be limited to brief periods of 5 or, at most, 10 minutes, or will the therapist allow longer phone consultations)?

- Does the person understand the steps to take and what resources are available in case of a crisis, emergency, or severe need?

- If the person or the treatment is to be used for teaching or related purposes, does the person adequately understand the nature, extent, and implications of such arrangements?

- Does the person demonstrate a sufficient understanding of the limitations of privacy, confidentiality, and privilege, especially in cases involving discretionary or mandatory reports by the therapist and potential legal actions the person may pursue in the context of therapist–patient sexual involvement?

- Does the person adequately understand the degree to which treatment notes and any other documents in the chart will be made available to the patient or the patient's attorney?

- Does the person have information or access to knowledge about options for filing formal complaints (e.g., licensing, malpractice, ethics, or criminal)?

- If the person has filed or is considering filing a lawsuit or other formal complaints against the previous therapist, is the person aware of how the procedures associated with such complaints may affect the therapy process?

Because each patient, therapist, and therapy is unique, it's crucial for the therapist to consider any relevant issues that the preceding items in this list may have missed or not covered. As the therapist tries to identify empathically with the person seeking treatment, what would the therapist wish to know if they were in the patient's position? What information would the person want to know that might significantly affect their decision about beginning therapy?

PART **V** RESOURCES
FOR REVIEWING
TREATMENT PLANS,
NOTES, AND CHARTS

Resource C

POINTS TO CONSIDER WHEN REVIEWING THE TREATMENT PLAN OF A PATIENT WITH A HISTORY OF SEXUAL INVOLVEMENT WITH A PREVIOUS THERAPIST

- Is the patient showing signs of improvement up to this point? What concerns have been effectively addressed? What significant issues remain unresolved? What, if any, new problems have come up?

- Have the patient's strengths, abilities, and resources—personal, familial, community, and setting—been evaluated? Is the current treatment plan appropriately incorporating and leveraging these strengths, abilities, and resources?

- Have issues of informed consent been adequately addressed, particularly concerning any recent changes in the assessment strategy or treatment planning?

- Are the patient's descriptions of sexual involvement with a therapist or any other matters raising concerns about mandatory or discretionary reporting? If so, have these concerns been appropriately addressed?

- Have potential risks for violence, abuse, or life-threatening behaviors concerning this patient been adequately assessed?

- To what degree, if at all, does the patient seem to be experiencing any of the following:

  ☐ impaired ability to trust (often focused on conflicts about dependence, control, and power)

  ☐ guilt or remorse

- ☐ shame
- ☐ ambivalence
- ☐ feelings of emptiness and isolation
- ☐ identity and boundary disturbances
- ☐ confusion around sexual behaviors
- ☐ lability of mood (particularly involving depression)
- ☐ suppressed rage
- ☐ increased suicidal risk
- ☐ cognitive dysfunction (especially in the areas of attention and concentration, frequently involving intrusive thoughts, unbidden images, flashbacks, and nightmares)

If so, are these issues adequately addressed in the treatment plan?

- Did the sexual involvement with the therapist result in a pregnancy?

- Is there any evidence that the patient has medical needs that are not being met? Are there any issues or concerns about the possibility of HIV, HPV, herpes, syphilis, hepatitis, gonorrhea, or any other sexually transmitted infections that need to be addressed?

- If other professionals (e.g., an attorney handling a malpractice suit against the previous therapist) are also providing services to the patient, are relevant issues related to the coordination of services, miscommunications, turf issues, lines of responsibility, and so on being adequately addressed?

- Do the chart notes and documentation adequately reflect the current state of assessment, treatment, and treatment planning?

- Have any treatment concerns emerged for which the therapist is not adequately competent or prepared? If so, have these concerns been sufficiently addressed through options such as supervision or consultation?

- Is the therapist experiencing, for whatever reasons, the type of reactions that might constitute countertransference, bias, or some other phenomenon that might distort, block, or otherwise interfere with providing adequate professional services? Reactions can include boredom and disinterest in the case, a propensity to blame the client, an overwhelming urge to control the patient, a wish or tendency to avoid contact with the patient, or extreme discomfort at the prospect that they might be called to testify in a malpractice suit against a fellow therapist. If so, have these reactions been adequately addressed (e.g., through consultation with a colleague)?

GUIDELINES FOR REVIEWING A PRIOR THERAPIST'S TREATMENT NOTES AND CHART MATERIALS

Clinicians who provide therapy or conduct forensic assessments in cases where therapist–patient sexual relationships are alleged typically perform a comprehensive review of previous treatment records. Unless the records are withheld or unavailable, this review is critical. Consider the following questions during the review process to ensure a complete evaluation:

- Do the records specify the referral source? Was the referral source contacted again?

- Do the records specify why the individual sought therapy?

- Was a mental status examination conducted, and are the results documented?

- Is there any mention of psychological tests or standardized assessment tools that were completed? If so, are the raw data, scoring sheets, and interpretations (including computerized scores or interpretations) available for you to review? Was the testing conducted in English or any other language? If the testing was not conducted in English, was any information provided about the norms that were used?

- Is the patient's physical or medical condition(s) and history mentioned?

- Is there any indication about whether the individual is or was suffering from any physical or medical condition?

- Was there any mention or indication of any factor(s) that might affect the ease, clarity, and effectiveness of communication? For example, was the client deaf or hard of hearing? Was the client completely fluent in and at ease speaking English? Did the client speak English with an accent? Did the client not speak English? If so, was the translation done by someone professionally trained to translate in clinical settings? Or was the translation done by one of the client's relatives or friends?

- Was a thorough history documented? Are any significant historical details overlooked?

- Are any records of previous assessments, treatments, hospitalizations, or other related information available for your review?

- Is there a documented diagnosis; if so, when was it first made? If it follows the *Diagnostic and Statistical Manual of Mental Disorders* (5th ed., text rev.; *DSM*; American Psychiatric Association, 2022), how were the criteria of the patient's condition evaluated? Be sure to check to see which edition of the *DSM* was used. Has the initial diagnosis been revised?

- Are there any indications of hallucinations, delusions, or similar phenomena? If so, when were they first noted, what additional assessment of such conditions was conducted, and how have they been addressed if at all? (Note that defense attorneys frequently assert that claims of sexual involvement are false and the result of delusions or the conditions noted in the questions that immediately follow.)

- Is any indication of an actual or potential psychosis documented?

- Is any indication of a factitious disorder documented?

- Was there any evidence of malingering or suboptimal effort on the part of the patient during their psychological or cognitive evaluation?

- Does the documentation include any indication that there was a treatment plan? If so, is there any indication that the effectiveness of the treatment plan was carefully monitored? In what ways was the treatment plan effective, ineffective, or harmful? Is there any indication that the treatment plan was ever revised in light of progress in therapy, new information, or other factors?

- Is there documentation of the patient's informed consent for treatment? If so, what specific treatments or procedures did the patient consent to?

- Did the therapist refer the patient to other professionals, facilities, or organizations for consultation, assessment, adjunctive treatment, or other purposes? If so, is there a record of the referral's outcomes?

- Is there any indication that the therapist issued or received requests for information from other professionals, facilities, or organizations regarding this patient? If so, are the requests accompanied by an appropriate waiver of confidentiality from the patient? Is it clear what information was sent to or received from others?

- Do the billing records appear to be clear and complete?

- Does the fee for service ever change? If so, do the records indicate the reason for the change?

- Are therapy notes and billing records available for all sessions? Were all sessions billed appropriately, or were there any instances where the patient was not billed?

- Were there third-party payment sources (e.g., private insurance or governmental plan)? What diagnosis (or diagnoses), session dates, and so forth were provided to the payment source, and is this information in accord with information elsewhere in the chart materials?

- Is there any indication of sexual attraction or feelings, discussion, or behavior on the part of either the patient or therapist?

- Is there any indication of texting, sexting, or interactions on social media or communication via social media direct messages?

- Is there any indication of physical contact between the therapist and the patient? If so, what kind of physical contact?

- Did meetings between therapist and patient ever occur outside the clinical consulting room? If so, what were the rationale and conditions? Were any sessions conducted by phone or videoconference?

- Is there any mention of transference or countertransference?

- To what extent was there a formal termination process?

- Why did the therapist and patient stop meeting? Which factors mentioned in the documentation are relevant to the termination of formal sessions or informal meetings between the therapist and patient?

- Does anything significant appear to be missing from the records available for your review?

PART **VI** RESOURCES ON PREPARING FOR DEPOSITION AND CROSS-EXAMINATION

TEN QUESTIONS TO HELP THERAPISTS PREPARE FOR DEPOSITION AND CROSS-EXAMINATION

1. Will the patient be present during the therapist's testimony, and if so, have concerns about the patient encountering the therapist in a different setting and listening to testimony been appropriately discussed and addressed?

2. Have relevant published works on the topic of therapist–patient sexual relationships—including research, theory, and related materials—been reviewed?

3. Is the therapist's curriculum vitae accurate, complete, and up to date?

4. Is the curriculum vitae sufficiently clear in demonstrating the therapist's education, training, and experience in providing assessment, therapeutic, and forensic services in the context of patients who have been sexually involved with a previous therapist, helping to establish a demonstrable level of competence or expertise? If not, can the therapist address any concerns regarding their competence or expertise in this area?

5. Have all chart notes and related documents been reviewed?

6. Have any of the therapist's documents (e.g., chart notes, billing records, assessment data) or other materials been subpoenaed? If so, have all issues related to the release of these documents and materials been adequately addressed and resolved (e.g., considering potential privilege protection)? If the therapist plans to bring the documents and materials, have they been appropriately located and secured?

7. Does the therapist have a realistic understanding of how much time their testimony may take so they can plan accordingly? For example, the therapist may be scheduled to testify Wednesday morning. The attorney calling the therapist to testify may have stressed that the direct examination will begin at 9:00 a.m. and should take at most an hour. The attorney estimates that the cross-examination will also take no more than an hour. So, the therapist plans to complete testimony by noon and see patients beginning at 1:30 in the afternoon. However, there may be long delays before the court is called to order Wednesday morning. Numerous objections, unexpected rulings, and several recesses may stretch the direct examination to two or three times the estimated length. The attorney conducting the cross-examination may question the therapist for literally 2 or 3 days. The possibility that the therapist may not be done with their testimony by Wednesday afternoon needs to be adequately discussed, and contingency plans need to be created.

8. Have all relevant parties established and adhered to payment arrangements for the therapist's deposition or trial testimony?

9. Is it advisable or beneficial for the therapist to seek the counsel of their attorney when summoned to testify as a witness in a case involving their current or former patient? In many instances, therapists rely on the guidance of the attorney who calls them to testify. However, because that attorney primarily represents the interests of another party, it may be wise for a therapist to consider consulting with an independent legal counsel. This can help address potential ethical and legal considerations that may arise.

10. Is the therapist aware of factors that may impact their testimony? For instance, can the therapist identify any strong feelings or other emotional reactions, biases, countertransference, or other personal factors that might interfere with their ability to provide clear, truthful, and undistorted testimony? If so, how can these be effectively addressed before the testimony?

Resource F

CROSS-EXAMINATION QUESTIONS FOR THERAPISTS WHO TESTIFY ABOUT A PATIENT'S SEXUAL INVOLVEMENT WITH A THERAPIST

Therapists providing clinical services to patients who allege sexual involvement with a prior therapist are likely to face an extensive and probing deposition and challenging cross-examination if a lawsuit goes to trial. This resource offers a set of review questions to help clinicians prepare. Reviewing these questions in advance will not only eliminate the element of surprise that occurs when a therapist encounters them for the first time while testifying under oath but also provide the witness with the opportunity to reflect on their meaning. This preview also allows the witness to examine relevant information, such as treatment records and pertinent publications, and consider these questions from various angles before offering their responses under oath. Thinking about these questions ahead of time can help the therapist ensure that the answers they provide when they testify are as clear, informed, accurate, and nondefensive as possible.

Reviewing these questions will not only help therapists prepare to testify in a specific case but also provide opportunities to rethink and reevaluate their work more generally. Considering these questions and their implications can help therapists identify and address weaknesses in their practice.

Although these questions are phrased for the subsequent therapist, they can also help other mental health witnesses (expert or fact), regardless of whether they are called by the patient's attorney, the previous therapist's attorney (i.e., the therapist alleged to have engaged in therapist–patient sexual activity), attorneys for other parties to the case (e.g., the previous therapist's supervisor or the hospital or managed care facility for which the previous therapist was working when the sexual involvement was alleged to have occurred), or by the court itself (e.g., when the court appoints a clinician to conduct an independent psychological assessment of the patient).

THE THERAPIST'S PREVIOUS WORK WITH PATIENTS WHO ALLEGE SEXUAL INVOLVEMENT

- How many patients have you seen clinically who have alleged that they were sexually involved with a former therapist?

- When you consider all the instances in which patients have alleged to you that they have been sexually involved with a previous therapist, how many instances of allegations were there that you finally concluded were valid? In how many instances did you conclude that the allegations were invalid? Were there any instances in which you could not reach a conclusion about the validity of the allegations?

- How do you assess the integrity of a patient's allegations? What specific types of evidence do you consider, and what factors influence your decision when determining whether the allegations are true or false? Please list the evidence you consider and the key elements of your reasoning.

THE THERAPIST'S KNOWLEDGE OF RELEVANT RESEARCH, THEORY, AND CURRENT PRACTICE

- Do you believe that a therapist working with a patient who is alleging therapist–patient sexual involvement needs to be adequately aware of the current research, theory, and practice relevant to therapist–patient sexual contact? (This question is a foundation for the questions that follow. If the therapist answers "no," it is likely that the attorney will elicit extensive testimony about the rationale and implications for this belief.)

- Are you adequately aware of the current research, theory, and practice relevant to therapist–patient sexual contact?

- Please summarize the most recent research studies in this area.

- Please summarize the most recent articles on theory in this area.

THE THERAPIST'S SOURCES OF KNOWLEDGE ABOUT THE PATIENT

- How many hours have you spent with the patient?

- Have you reviewed all relevant background documents? Please list those documents that you have reviewed. Would these include
  - prior medical records,
  - prior records of psychological assessment or treatment,
  - records of any hospitalizations,
  - school records,
  - prior records of employment, or
  - depositions and other legal documents?

- In conducting your assessment of this patient, providing therapy to this patient, preparing to testify, or at any other time, have you ever tried to contact or interview any family member, friend, or acquaintance of this patient?

- Have you ever tried to contact or interview teachers, employers, coworkers, or other people involved in this patient's education or work?

- Have you attempted to reach out to or conduct an interview with the former therapist whom the patient alleges they had sex with?

- Have you made any effort to contact or interview any health care or mental health care professional who has provided assessment, treatment, consultation, or other services to the patient?

- Aside from those individuals previously mentioned, have you made any effort to contact or interview anyone else who might have information relevant to your assessment of the patient, the therapy you provided, or your testimony here today?

THE THERAPIST'S USE OF OR RELIANCE ON STANDARDIZED PSYCHOLOGICAL TESTS

- Was your therapy with this patient guided by an assessment that included standardized psychological tests, regardless of whether you personally administered, scored, or interpreted the tests?

- For each test, what is the reliability and validity when the test is used with this population (i.e., people who allege sexual involvement with a prior therapist)?

- Did the assessment include the use of embedded or stand-alone measures of effort?

- Are you aware of any standardized tests that can reliably indicate whether a patient has been sexually involved with a prior therapist?

- Are you aware of any research indicating that psychological test results can be misleading if interpreted in the absence of an adequate history?

- What aspects of this patient's characteristics and personal history were relevant to properly interpreting the psychological tests?

FINANCIAL CONCERNS

- How much are you charging for your testimony in this case?

- When did you first discuss financial arrangements (e.g., how much the patient would pay per session) with the patient? What was the nature of those original arrangements? Were those arrangements part of the informed consent?

- Have the financial arrangements been changed in any way? If so, when and how?

- Have the financial arrangements, including changes, been fully documented?

- Did you, the patient, or any other relevant person ever depart in any way from these financial arrangements?

- Under these financial arrangements, how much money have you earned— whether or not the money has been paid to you—for your time and work with this patient?

- Up to now, how much money, if any, has been paid to you?

- Currently, how much is owed to you? (Significant amounts will probably form the basis of numerous subsequent questions addressing issues, such as the therapist allowing a substantial debt to accumulate and how the likelihood of payment of this debt might hinge on the outcome of the trial, which in turn might be affected by the therapist's testimony. In the latter instance, the therapist's possible bias is explored; the cross-examining attorney's questions may make clear that the therapist's testimony may significantly influence whether the therapist receives payment of money owed to them.)

- Have you ever sought a lien for any money the patient owes you?

- Have any of the attorneys in this case or those acting on the attorney's behalf offered you any money for your services or other reasons?

- Will you receive any money that is contingent on the outcome of this case?

COMPLIANCE WITH SUBPOENA DUCES TECUM

The three sets of questions in this section are taken verbatim from Pope et al. (2006).

- Have you complied fully with each and every item that the subpoena asked you to produce? Are there any items that you did not make available?

- Were any of these documents altered in any way? Were any of them recopied, erased, written over, enhanced, edited, or added to in any way since the time each was originally created? Are the photocopies made available true and exact replicas of the original documents without any revision?

- Have any documents falling within the scope of the subpoena or otherwise relevant to the case been lost, stolen, misplaced, destroyed, or thrown away? Are any documents you made, collected, handled, or received that are within the scope of this subpoena or otherwise relevant to the case absent from the documents made available to me? (p. 173)

THE THERAPIST'S FORENSIC EXPERIENCE WHEN THERAPIST-PATIENT SEX WAS AT ISSUE

- Have you ever participated in civil, criminal, licensing, or any other forums in which allegations of therapist–patient sexual contact were at issue?

- How many such cases involved patients to whom you had personally provided professional services?

- In how many such cases did you appear as a witness called by the plaintiff?

- In how many such cases did you appear as a witness called by the defense?

- In how many such cases did you appear in some other capacity than as a witness called by the plaintiff or defense?

- In how many such cases have you been allowed to testify as an expert witness (rather than in some other capacity, such as a percipient or fact witness)?

PART **VII** RESOURCE FOR
SUBPOENAS
AND COMPELLED
TESTIMONY

Resource G

STRATEGIES FOR PRIVATE PRACTITIONERS COPING WITH SUBPOENAS OR COMPELLED TESTIMONY FOR CLIENT/PATIENT RECORDS OR TEST DATA OR TEST MATERIALS[1]

COMMITTEE ON LEGAL ISSUES, AMERICAN PSYCHOLOGICAL ASSOCIATION

In response to a large number of inquiries by psychologists faced with subpoenas or compelled court testimony concerning Client/Patient records or test data, manuals, protocols, and other test information, the American Psychological Association's (APA) Committee on Legal Issues prepared this article. It identifies legal issues that may arise from such subpoenas and similar legal demands, and it suggests strategies that might be considered in the event such a subpoena or demand is received. This document is not intended to establish any standards of care or conduct for practitioners; rather, it addresses this general question: What strategies may be available to psychologists in private practice for responding to subpoenas or compelled court testimony concerning Client/Patient records, test data, test manuals, test protocols, or other test information?

All citizens are required, as a general principle of law, to provide information necessary for deciding issues before a court. From the perspective of the legal system, the more relevant the available information is to the trier of fact (i.e., judge or jury), the fairer the decision. Statutes, rules of civil and

[1]Adapted from "Strategies for Private Practitioners Coping With Subpoenas or Compelled Testimony for Client/Patient Records or Test Data or Test Materials," by the Committee on Legal Issues, American Psychological Association, 2016, *Professional Psychology: Research and Practice*, *47*(1), pp. 1–11 (https://doi.org/ 10.1037/pro0000063). Copyright 2016 by the American Psychological Association.

criminal procedure, and rules of evidence have established the procedures for the transmittal of such information. In order to obtain this material, the court may issue *subpoenas* (legal commands to appear to provide testimony) or *subpoenas duces tecum* (legal commands to appear and bring along specific documents). Alternatively, the court may issue a court order to provide testimony or produce documents. A subpoena issued by an attorney under court rules, requesting testimony or documents, even if not signed by a judge, requires a timely response, but it may be modified or quashed (i.e., made void or invalid).

It is important to differentiate responding to a subpoena from disclosing confidential information. Unless the issuing attorney or court excuses the psychologist, it will be necessary to respond to a subpoena, that is, to be at a particular place at a particular time (with records if the subpoena is a subpoena duces tecum). Responding to the subpoena, however, does not necessarily entail disclosing confidential information. In order to disclose confidential information, a psychologist will need to ensure that the conditions for disclosing confidential information, such as the Client/Patient's consent or a judge's order or other legal mandate, are met, in addition to having a valid subpoena. Thus, while a subpoena requires a response, a subpoena alone will generally not be sufficient to warrant a disclosure of confidential information. However, once a court order for testimony or documents is issued and any attempt (made in a timely manner) to have the court vacate or modify its order has been unsuccessful, a psychologist may be held in contempt of court if he or she fails to comply.

The demands of the legal system sometimes conflict with the responsibility of psychologists to maintain the confidentiality of Client/Patient records. This responsibility arises from tenets of good clinical practice, ethical standards, professional licensing laws, and other applicable statutes and legal precedent. In many contexts, the Client/Patient material generated in the course of a professional relationship may also fall under an evidentiary privilege, which protects such information from judicial scrutiny. Most state and federal jurisdictions recognize a patient privilege that allows the Client/Patient to prevent confidential material conveyed to a psychologist from being communicated to others in legal settings although there are variations from state to state and between state and federal definitions. In most jurisdictions, the privilege belongs to the Client/Patient, not to the therapist. The psychologist has a responsibility to maintain confidentiality and to assert the psychotherapist–patient privilege unless the Client/Patient has explicitly waived privilege or signed a valid release, unless a legally recognized exception to privilege exists, or unless the court orders the psychologist to turn over the Client/Patient's information.

The clinical record, any separately kept psychotherapy notes, Client/Patient information forms, billing records, and other such information usually may be turned over to the court with appropriate authorization by the Client/Patient or with a court order. (Psychologists who need to comply with the Health Insurance Portability and Accountability Act of 1996 (HIPAA) would need a HIPAA-compliant authorization form to release such information, and a separate authorization for release of psychotherapy notes. The risk of disclosure through subpoena or court order should be disclosed to Client/Patients in the informed consent document and discussion.) Psychological test material and test data can present a more complicated situation. Although a Client/Patient's test data may have to be released in response to a subpoena, the disclosure of test materials (i.e., manuals, instruments, protocols, and test questions) may require the additional safeguard of a court order because the inappropriate disclosure of test materials may seriously impair the security and threaten the validity of the test and its value as a measurement tool.

Psychologists have numerous ethical, professional, and legal obligations that touch on the release of Client/Patient records, test data, and other information in the legal context. Many such obligations may favor disclosure, including, in particular, the general obligation of all citizens to give truthful and complete testimony in courts of law when subpoenaed to do so. But there are often conflicting duties and principles that favor withholding such information. These may include obligations to (a) Client/Patients or other individuals who receive treatment and/or are assessed or administered psychological tests (e.g., privileged or confidential communications that may include Client/Patient responses to test items), (b) the public (e.g., to avoid public dissemination of test items, questions, protocols, or other test information that could adversely affect the integrity and continued validity of tests), (c) test publishers (e.g., contractual obligations between the psychologist and test publishers not to disclose test information; obligations under the copyright laws), and (d) other third parties (e.g., employers). It merits mention that a special type of third-party obligation may arise in forensic contexts: If, for example, a psychologist performed work for an attorney, it is important to investigate whether that work is protected from disclosure under the attorney work product privilege. The aforementioned obligations may, at times, conflict with one another. Psychologists must identify and seek to reconcile their obligations. For more on these obligations, see APA's *Ethical Principles of Psychologists and Code of Conduct* (American Psychological Association, 2017), hereinafter referred to as the APA Ethics Code (see Appendix A).

There are specific settings (e.g., educational, institutional, employment) in which the legal or ethical obligations of psychologists as they relate to disclosure of Client/Patient records or test information present special problems.

This article does not purport to address disclosure issues in these special contexts, nor does it attempt to resolve dilemmas faced by psychologists in reconciling legal and ethical obligations.

STRATEGIES FOR DEALING WITH SUBPOENAS

Determine Whether the Request for Information Carries the Force of Law

It must first be determined whether a psychologist has, in fact, received a legally valid demand for disclosure of sensitive test data and Client/Patient records. If a demand is not legally enforceable for any reason, then the psychologist has no legal obligation to comply with it and may have no legal obligation even to respond. A subpoena to produce documents generally must allow sufficient time to respond to the demand and provide for some time within which the opposing side may move to quash such a demand. Without this allowed time period, the subpoena may not be valid. Even a demand that claims to be legally enforceable may not be. For example, the court issuing the subpoena may not have jurisdiction over the psychologist or his or her records (e.g., a subpoena issued in one state may not be legally binding on a psychologist residing and working in a different state). Or, the subpoena may not have been properly served on the psychologist (e.g., some states may require service in person or by certified mail or that a subpoena for such records be accompanied by a special court order). It is advisable that a psychologist consult with an attorney in making such a determination.[2]

---

[2]It is important to recognize that the client's attorney, or the attorney who issues the subpoena, is not the psychologist's attorney and may represent interests different from those of the psychologist. Thus, the psychologist may not be able to rely upon the information provided by that attorney. Psychologists can find attorneys with experience representing psychologists via their states' bar associations, their states' psychological association, colleagues, and local attorneys.

Fees for consultation with or representation by an attorney may be substantial. If consultation with an attorney becomes necessary to protect the interests and privileges of the client, then the practitioner may wish to clarify with his or her client who will be responsible for such legal fees. In some cases, malpractice carriers will authorize legal consultation free of charge. During an initial consultation, psychologists should ask an attorney the following questions before hiring him or her: (a) How many psychologists or other medical professionals has the attorney represented? (b) Is the attorney familiar with the state's psychology licensing statute and ethical code? (c) How many psychologists or other medical professionals has the attorney represented in licensing actions/ethical complaints? (d) Is the attorney familiar with the federal HIPAA law and the state's confidentiality statutes? In addition, the psychologist should not hesitate to ask other relevant questions about fees, retainers, and the like.

If the psychologist concludes that the demand is legally valid, then some formal response to the attorney or court will be required—either compliance with or opposition to the demand, in whole or in part. A psychologist's obligations in responding to a valid subpoena are not necessarily the same as those under a court order (see section titled File a Motion to Quash the Subpoena or File a Protective Order). The next step, in most cases, may involve contacting the psychologist's Client/Patient. However, the psychologist may wish to consider grounds for opposing or limiting production of the demanded information before contacting the Client/Patient so that the Client/Patient can more fully understand his or her options (see section titled Possible Grounds for Opposing or Limiting Production of Client/Patient Records or Test Data).

Contact the Client/Patient

The Client/Patient to whom requested records pertain often has a legally protected interest in preserving the confidentiality of the records. If, therefore, a psychologist receives a subpoena or advance notice that he or she may be required to divulge Client/Patient records or test data, the psychologist may, when appropriate, discuss the implications of the demand with the Client/Patient (or his or her legal guardian). Also, when appropriate and with the Client/Patient's valid consent, the psychologist may consult with the Client/Patient's attorney. The discussion with the Client/Patient will inform the Client/Patient which information has been demanded, the purpose of the demand, the entities or individuals to whom the information is to be provided, and the possible scope of further disclosure by those entities or individuals. Following such a discussion, a legally competent Client/Patient or the Client/Patient's legal guardian may choose to consent to production of the data. Generally, it is legally required to have such consent in writing, for clarity and if there is a need for documentation in the future. Written consent may avoid future conflicts or legal entanglements with the Client/Patient over the release of confidential tests or other records pertaining to the Client/Patient. The Client/Patient's consent may not, however, resolve the potential confidentiality claims of third parties (such as test publishers). For more information, see APA Ethics Code, Ethical Standards, Section 4 (American Psychological Association, 2017), and *Standards for Educational and Psychological Testing* (American Educational Research Association, American Psychological Association, & National Council on Measurement in Education, 2014).

It also merits emphasis to a Client/Patient that when agreeing to release information requested in a subpoena, he or she cannot specify or limit which information is released, rather, the entire record (e.g., psychotherapy notes, billing records administrative notes) will be available. The scope of the release may be the subject of negotiation among attorneys, however, and if the psychologist believes that a release would harm the Client/Patient, the psychologist should voice his or her concerns and object to the release on that basis.

Negotiate With the Requester

If a Client/Patient does not consent to release of the requested information, the psychologist (often through counsel) may seek to prevent disclosure through discussions with legal counsel for the requesting party. The psychologist's position in such discussions may be bolstered by legal arguments against disclosure, including the psychologist's duties under rules regarding psychotherapist–patient privilege. These rules often allow the psychologist to assert privilege on behalf of the Client/Patient in the absence of a specific release or court order. (Some possible arguments are outlined in the section titled Possible Grounds for Opposing or Limiting Production of Client/Patient Records or Test Data.) Such negotiations may explore whether there are ways to achieve the requesting party's objectives without divulging confidential information, for example, through disclosure of nonconfidential materials or submission of an affidavit by the psychologist disclosing nonconfidential information. Negotiation may also be used as a strategy to avoid compelled testimony in court or by deposition. In short, negotiation can be explored as a possible means of avoiding the wholesale release of confidential test or Client/Patient information—release that may not be in the best interests of the Client/Patient, the public, or the profession and that may not even be relevant to the issues before the court. Such an option could be explored in consultation with the psychologist's attorney or the Client/Patient's attorney.

File a Motion to Quash the Subpoena or File a Protective Order

If negotiation is not successful, it may be necessary to file a motion for relief from the obligations imposed by the demand for production of the confidential records. In many jurisdictions, the possible motions include a motion to quash the subpoena, in whole or in part, or a motion for a protective order. Filing such a motion may require the assistance of counsel, representing either the psychologist or the psychologist's Client/Patient.

Courts are generally more receptive to a motion to quash or a motion for a protective order if it is filed by the Client/Patient about whom information is sought (who would be defending his or her own interests) rather than by a psychologist who, in essence, would be seeking to protect the rights of the

Client/Patient or other third parties. The psychologist may wish to determine initially whether the Client/Patient's lawyer is inclined to seek to quash a subpoena or to seek a protective order and, if so, may wish to provide assistance to the Client/Patient's attorney in this regard. If the Client/Patient has refused to consent to disclosure of the information, his or her attorney may be willing to take the lead in opposing the subpoena.

A *motion to quash* is a formal application made to a court or judge for purposes of having a subpoena vacated or declared invalid. Grounds may exist for asserting that the subpoena or request for testimony should be quashed, in whole or in part. For example, the information sought may be protected by the therapist–Client/Patient privilege and therefore may not be subject to discovery, or it may not be relevant to the issues before the court (see section titled Possible Grounds for Opposing or Limiting Production of Client/Patient Records or Test Data). This strategy may be used alone or in combination with a motion for a protective order.

A *motion for a protective order* anticipates production of material responsive to the subpoena but seeks an order or decree from the court that protects against the untoward consequences of disclosing information. A protective order can be tailored to meet the legitimate interests of the Client/Patient and of third parties such as test publishers and the public. The focus of this strategy first and foremost is to prevent or limit those to whom produced information may be disclosed and the use of sensitive Client/Patient and test information. The protective order—and the motion—may include any of the elements listed below.

Generally, the motion may state that the psychologist is ethically obligated not to produce the confidential records or test data or to testify about them unless compelled to do so by the court or with the consent of the Client/Patient. It may include a request that the court consider the psychologist's obligations to adhere to federal requirements (e.g., HIPAA) and to protect the interests of the Client/Patient, the interests of third parties (e.g., test publishers or others), and the public's interest in preserving the integrity and continued validity of the tests themselves. This may help sensitize the court to the potential adverse effects of dissemination. The motion might also attempt to provide suggestions, such as the following, to the court about ways to minimize the adverse consequences of disclosure if the court is inclined to require production at all:

1. Suggest that the court direct the psychologist to provide test data only to another appropriately qualified professional designated by the court or by the party seeking such information. The manual for the test should specify the credentials of the professional who is qualified to use it.

2. Suggest that the court limit the use of Client/Patient records or test data to prevent wide dissemination. For example, the court might order that the information be delivered to the court, be kept under seal, be used solely for the purposes of the litigation, and that all copies of the data be returned to the psychologist under seal after the litigation is terminated. The order might also provide that the requester must prevent or limit the disclosure of the information to third parties.

3. Suggest that the court limit the categories of information that must be produced. For example, Client/Patient records may contain confidential information about a third party, such as a spouse, who may have independent interests in maintaining confidentiality, and such data may be of minimal or no relevance to the issues before the court. The court should limit its production order to exclude such information.

4. Suggest that the court determine for itself, through in camera proceedings (i.e., a nonpublic hearing or a review by the judge in chambers), whether the use of the Client/Patient records or test data is relevant to the issues before the court or whether it might be insulated from disclosure, in whole or in part, by the therapist–Client/Patient privilege or another privilege (e.g., attorney–Client/Patient privilege).

5. Suggest that the court deny or limit the demand because it is unduly burdensome on the psychologist (see, e.g., Federal Rule of Civil Procedure 45(c)).

6. Suggest that the court shield from production "psychotherapy notes" if the psychologist keeps separate psychotherapy notes as defined by the Privacy Rule (see Security and Privacy, 2015). See rule excerpts in Appendix B.

PSYCHOLOGISTS' TESTIMONY

If a psychologist is asked to disclose confidential information during questioning at a deposition, he or she may refuse to answer the question only if the information is privileged. If there is a reasonable basis for asserting a privilege, the psychologist may refuse to provide test data or Client/Patient records until so ordered by the court. A psychologist who refuses to answer questions without a reasonable basis may be penalized by the court, including the obligation to pay the requesting parties' costs and fees in obtaining court enforcement of the subpoena. For these reasons, it is advisable that a psychologist be represented by his or her own counsel at the deposition. A lawyer may advise the psychologist, on the record, when a question seeks confidential information; such on-the-record advice will help protect the psychologist from the adverse legal consequences of erroneous disclosures or erroneous refusals to disclose.

Similarly, if the request for confidential information arises for the first time during courtroom testimony, the psychologist may assert a privilege and refuse to answer unless directed to do so by the court. The law in this area is somewhat unsettled. Thus, it may be advisable for him or her to consult an attorney before testifying.

POSSIBLE GROUNDS FOR OPPOSING OR LIMITING PRODUCTION OF CLIENT/PATIENT RECORDS OR TEST DATA

The following options may or may not be available under the facts of a particular case and/or a particular jurisdiction for resisting a demand to produce confidential information, records, or test data (see Appendix C):

1. The court does not have jurisdiction over the psychologist, the Client/Patient records, or the test data, or the psychologist did not receive a legally sufficient demand (e.g., improper service) for production of records or test data testimony.

2. The psychologist does not have custody or control of the records or test data that are sought, because, for example, they belong not to the psychologist but to his or her employer.

3. The therapist–Client/Patient privilege insulates the records or test data from disclosure. The rationale for the privilege, recognized in many states, is that the openness necessary for effective therapy requires that Client/Patients have an expectation that all records of therapy, contents of therapeutic disclosures, and test data will remain confidential. Disclosure would be a serious invasion of the Client/Patient's privacy. The psychologist is under an ethical obligation to protect the client's reasonable expectations of confidentiality. See APA Ethics Code, Ethical Standards, Section 4 (American Psychological Association, 2017). There are important exceptions to this protection that negate the privilege. For example, if the Client/former client is a party to the litigation and has raised his/her mental state as an issue in the proceeding, the client may have waived the psychotherapist–patient privilege. This varies by jurisdiction with most jurisdictions holding a broad patient–litigant exception to privilege, with a few construing the patient–litigant exception much more narrowly. It is important that the psychologist be aware of the law in the relevant jurisdiction, because this may ultimately control the issue about

release of (otherwise) confidential client information. In this circumstance, the fact that a client who is a party to a legal case does not want to consent to release of information may not ultimately be dispositive on the issue. In such a case, the psychologist should discuss the issue of potential patient–litigant exception with the client's attorney, to determine if the records will need to be turned over due to the exception and to obtain any needed authorizations from the client.[3]

4. The information sought is not relevant to the issues before the court, or the scope of the demand for information is overbroad in reaching information not relevant to the issues before the court, including irrelevant information pertaining to third parties such as a spouse.

5. Public dissemination of test information such as manuals, protocols, and so forth may harm the public interest because it may affect responses of future test populations. This effect could result in the loss of valuable assessment tools to the detriment of both the public and the profession of psychology.

6. Test publishers have an interest in the protection of test information, and the psychologist may have a contractual or other legal obligation (e.g., copyright laws) not to disclose such information. Such contractual claims, coupled with concerns about test data devolving into the public domain and thereby, diminishing its usefulness to the courts, may justify issuance of a protective order against dissemination of a test instrument or protocols.[4]

---

[3]A psychologist's obligation to maintain confidentiality may not apply under certain legally recognized exceptions to the therapist–patient privilege, including, but not limited to, situations such as the following: when child or elder abuse is involved; cases involving involuntary commitment evaluations; court-ordered evaluations; when clients raise their emotional condition as a basis for a legal claim or defense; or when the client presents an imminent danger to himself or herself or the community. Exceptions may depend on jurisdiction and the facts of a particular situation. Thus, the most prudent course of action may be for the psychologist to consult with an attorney.

[4]Most test publishers have policies that address the disclosure of test data and materials. Very often, such policies can be found on a test publisher's website, along with other information such as terms of purchasing psychological tests, the publisher's position on legal aspects of disclosing test data and test materials and contact information for the test publisher's privacy officer or general counsel. Reviewing a particular test publisher's website can be very helpful when psychologists are considering disclosing test data or test materials, especially when the disclosure potentially involves nonpsychologists. Psychologists should be aware that the information on test publisher websites may or may not be consistent with APA policy, may not reflect exceptions that apply in certain states, and APA takes no position on the accuracy of legal statements or claims found on such websites.

7. Psychologists have an ethical obligation to protect the integrity and security of test information and data including protecting the intellectual property (copyright) and unauthorized test disclosure, and to avoid misuse of assessment techniques and data. Psychologists are also ethically obligated to take reasonable steps to prevent others from misusing such information. See APA Ethics Code, Ethical Standards, Section 2 (American Psychological Association, 2017).

8. Refer to ethical and legal obligations of psychologists as provided for under ethics codes; professional standards; state, federal, or local laws; or regulatory agencies.

9. Some court rules allow the party receiving the subpoena to object to the subpoena's demand or ask that the demand be limited on the basis that it imposes an undue burden on the recipient (see, e.g., Rule 45(c) of the Federal Rules of Civil Procedure, 2014).

10. Ultimately, the judge's ruling controls in a court. Psychologists who are not violating human rights and who take reasonable steps to follow Standard 1.02 of the APA Ethics Code and inform the Court of their requirements under the APA Ethics Code will not be subject to disciplinary procedures for complying with a court order directing to produce information.

Appendix A

EXCERPTS FROM THE AMERICAN PSYCHOLOGICAL ASSOCIATION'S *ETHICAL PRINCIPLES OF PSYCHOLOGISTS AND CODE OF CONDUCT*[1]

SECTION 1: RESOLVING ETHICAL ISSUES

1.02 Conflicts Between Ethics and Law, Regulations, or Other Governing Legal Authority

If psychologists' ethical responsibilities conflict with law, regulations, or other governing legal authority, psychologists clarify the nature of the conflict, make known their commitment to the Ethics Code, and take reasonable steps to resolve the conflict consistent with the General Principles and Ethical Standards of the Ethics Code. Under no circumstances may this standard be used to justify or defend violating human rights.

SECTION 2: COMPETENCE

2.01 Boundaries of Competence

(a) Psychologists provide services, teach, and conduct research with populations and in areas only within the boundaries of their competence, based on their education, training, supervised experience, consultation, study, or professional experience.

---

[1]From *Ethical Principles of Psychologists and Code of Conduct* (pp. 4–5, 7–9, 12–14), by the American Psychological Association, 2017 (https://www.apa.org/ethics/code/ethics-code-2017.pdf). Copyright 2017 by the American Psychological Association.

(b) Where scientific or professional knowledge in the discipline of psychology establishes that an understanding of factors associated with age, gender, gender identity, race, ethnicity, culture, national origin, religion, sexual orientation, disability, language, or socioeconomic status is essential for effective implementation of their services or research, psychologists have or obtain the training, experience, consultation, or supervision necessary to ensure the competence of their services, or they make appropriate referrals, except as provided in Standard 2.02, Providing Services in Emergencies.

(c) Psychologists planning to provide services, teach, or conduct research involving populations, areas, techniques, or technologies new to them undertake relevant education, training, supervised experience, consultation, or study.

(d) When psychologists are asked to provide services to individuals for whom appropriate mental health services are not available and for which psychologists have not obtained the competence necessary, psychologists with closely related prior training or experience may provide such services in order to ensure that services are not denied if they make a reasonable effort to obtain the competence required by using relevant research, training, consultation, or study.

(e) In those emerging areas in which generally recognized standards for preparatory training do not yet exist, psychologists nevertheless take reasonable steps to ensure the competence of their work and to protect clients/patients, students, supervisees, research participants, organizational clients, and others from harm.

(f) When assuming forensic roles, psychologists are or become reasonably familiar with the judicial or administrative rules governing their roles.

SECTION 4: PRIVACY AND CONFIDENTIALITY

4.01 Maintaining Confidentiality

Psychologists have a primary obligation and take reasonable precautions to protect confidential information obtained through or stored in any medium, recognizing that the extent and limits of confidentiality may be regulated by law or established by institutional rules or professional or scientific relationship. (See also Standard 2.05, Delegation of Work to Others.)

4.02 Discussing the Limits of Confidentiality

(a) Psychologists discuss with persons (including, to the extent feasible, persons who are legally incapable of giving informed consent and their legal representatives) and organizations with whom they establish a scientific or professional relationship (1) the relevant limits of confidentiality and (2) the foreseeable uses of the information generated through their psychological activities. (See also Standard 3.10, Informed Consent.)

(b) Unless it is not feasible or is contraindicated, the discussion of confidentiality occurs at the outset of the relationship and thereafter as new circumstances may warrant.

(c) Psychologists who offer services, products, or information via electronic transmission inform clients/patients of the risks to privacy and limits of confidentiality.

4.04 Minimizing Intrusions on Privacy

(a) Psychologists include in written and oral reports and consultations, only information germane to the purpose for which the communication is made.

(b) Psychologists discuss confidential information obtained in their work only for appropriate scientific or professional purposes and only with persons clearly concerned with such matters.

4.05 Disclosures

(a) Psychologists may disclose confidential information with the appropriate consent of the organizational client, the individual client/patient, or another legally authorized person on behalf of the client/patient unless prohibited by law.

(b) Psychologists disclose confidential information without the consent of the individual only as mandated by law, or where permitted by law for a valid purpose such as to (1) provide needed professional services; (2) obtain appropriate professional consultations; (3) protect the client/patient, psychologist, or others from harm; or (4) obtain payment for services from a client/patient, in which instance disclosure is limited to the minimum that is necessary to achieve the purpose. (See also Standard 6.04e, Fees and Financial Arrangements.)

SECTION 6: RECORD KEEPING AND FEES

6.01 Documentation of Professional and Scientific Work and Maintenance of Records

Psychologists create, and to the extent the records are under their control, maintain, disseminate, store, retain, and dispose of records and data relating to their professional and scientific work in order to (1) facilitate provision of services later by them or by other professionals, (2) allow for replication of research design and analyses, (3) meet institutional requirements, (4) ensure accuracy of billing and payments, and (5) ensure compliance with law. (See also Standard 4.01, Maintaining Confidentiality.)

6.02 Maintenance, Dissemination, and Disposal of Confidential Records of Professional and Scientific Work

(a) Psychologists maintain confidentiality in creating, storing, accessing, transferring, and disposing of records under their control, whether these are written, automated, or in any other medium. (See also Standards 4.01, Maintaining Confidentiality, and 6.01, Documentation of Professional and Scientific Work and Maintenance of Records.)

(b) If confidential information concerning recipients of psychological services is entered into databases or systems of records available to persons whose access has not been consented to by the recipient, psychologists use coding or other techniques to avoid the inclusion of personal identifiers.

(c) Psychologists make plans in advance to facilitate the appropriate transfer and to protect the confidentiality of records and data in the event of psychologists' withdrawal from positions or practice. (See also Standards 3.12, Interruption of Psychological Services, and 10.09, Interruption of Therapy.)

SECTION 9: ASSESSMENT

9.01 Bases for Assessments

(a) Psychologists base the opinions contained in their recommendations, reports, and diagnostic or evaluative statements, including forensic testimony, on information and techniques sufficient to substantiate their findings. (See also Standard 2.04, Bases for Scientific and Professional Judgments.)

(b) Except as noted in 9.01c, psychologists provide opinions of the psychological characteristics of individuals only after they have conducted an examination of the individuals adequate to support their statements or conclusions. When, despite reasonable efforts, such an examination is not practical, psychologists document the efforts they made and the result of those efforts, clarify the probable impact of their limited information on the reliability and validity of their opinions, and appropriately limit the nature and extent of their conclusions or recommendations. (See also Standards 2.01, Boundaries of Competence, and 9.06, Interpreting Assessment Results.)

(c) When psychologists conduct a record review or provide consultation or supervision and an individual examination is not warranted or necessary for the opinion, psychologists explain this and the sources of information on which they based their conclusions and recommendations.

9.02 Use of Assessments

(a) Psychologists administer, adapt, score, interpret, or use assessment techniques, interviews, tests, or instruments in a manner and for purposes that are appropriate in light of the research on or evidence of the usefulness and proper application of the techniques.

(b) Psychologists use assessment instruments whose validity and reliability have been established for use with members of the population tested. When such validity or reliability has not been established, psychologists describe the strengths and limitations of test results and interpretation.

(c) Psychologists use assessment methods that are appropriate to an individual's language preference and competence, unless the use of an alternative language is relevant to the assessment issues.

9.04 Release of Test Data

(a) The term *test data* refers to raw and scaled scores, client/patient responses to test questions or stimuli, and psychologists' notes and recordings concerning client/patient statements and behavior during an examination. Those portions of test materials that include client/patient responses are included in the definition of *test data*. Pursuant to a client/patient release, psychologists provide test data to the client/patient or other persons identified in the release. Psychologists may refrain from releasing test data to protect a client/patient or others from substantial harm or misuse or misrepresentation of the data or the test, recognizing that in many instances release of confidential information under these circumstances is regulated by law. (See also Standard 9.11, Maintaining Test Security.)

(b) In the absence of a client/patient release, psychologists provide test data only as required by law or court order.

9.06 Interpreting Assessment Results

When interpreting assessment results, including automated interpretations, psychologists take into account the purpose of the assessment as well as the various test factors, test-taking abilities, and other characteristics of the person being assessed, such as situational, personal, linguistic, and cultural differences, that might affect psychologists' judgments or reduce the accuracy of their interpretations. They indicate any significant limitations of their interpretations. (See also Standards 2.01b and c, Boundaries of Competence, and 3.01, Unfair Discrimination.)

9.07 Assessment by Unqualified Persons

Psychologists do not promote the use of psychological assessment techniques by unqualified persons, except when such use is conducted for training purposes with appropriate supervision. (See also Standard 2.05, Delegation of Work to Others.)

9.09 Test Scoring and Interpretation Services

(a) Psychologists who offer assessment or scoring services to other professionals accurately describe the purpose, norms, validity, reliability, and applications of the procedures and any special qualifications applicable to their use.

(b) Psychologists select scoring and interpretation services (including automated services) on the basis of evidence of the validity of the program and procedures as well as on other appropriate considerations. (See also Standard 2.01b and c, Boundaries of Competence.)

(c) Psychologists retain responsibility for the appropriate application, interpretation, and use of assessment instruments, whether they score and interpret such tests themselves or use automated or other services.

9.11 Maintaining Test Security

The term *test materials* refers to manuals, instruments, protocols, and test questions or stimuli and does not include *test data* as defined in Standard 9.04, Release of Test Data. Psychologists make reasonable efforts to maintain the integrity and security of test materials and other assessment techniques consistent with law and contractual obligations, and in a manner that permits adherence to this Ethics Code.

Appendix B

FEDERAL RULES AND REGULATIONS

EXCERPT FROM CODE OF FEDERAL REGULATIONS (U.S. DEPARTMENT OF HEALTH AND HUMAN SERVICES)[1]

Title 45–Public Welfare
Subtitle A–Department of Health and Human Services
Part 164–Security and Privacy
Subpart E–Privacy of Individually Identifiable Health Information
§164.501 Definitions
As used in this subpart, the following terms have the following meanings:

Psychotherapy notes means notes recorded (in any medium) by a health care provider who is a mental health professional documenting or analyzing the contents of conversation during a private counseling session or a group, joint, or family counseling session and that are separated from the rest of the individual's medical record. Psychotherapy notes excludes medication prescription and monitoring, counseling session start and stop times, the modalities and frequencies of treatment furnished, results of clinical tests, and any summary of the following items: Diagnosis, functional status, the treatment plan, symptoms, prognosis, and progress to date.

---

[1]From *Subpart E—Privacy of Individually Identifiable Health Information*, by the U.S. Department of Health and Human Services (pp. 643–646), 2023 (https://www.govinfo.gov/content/pkg/CFR-2023-title45-vol2/pdf/CFR-2023-title45-vol2-sec164-501.pdf). In the public domain.

EXCERPT FROM FEDERAL RULES OF CIVIL PROCEDURE (COMMITTEE ON THE JUDICIARY, HOUSE OF REPRESENTATIVES)[2]

Title VI. Trials

Rule 45. Subpoena

(d) Protecting a Person Subject to a Subpoena; Enforcement.

    (1) *Avoiding Undue Burden or Expense; Sanctions.* A party or attorney responsible for issuing and serving a subpoena must take reasonable steps to avoid imposing undue burden or expense on a person subject to the subpoena. The court for the district where compliance is required must enforce this duty and impose an appropriate sanction—which may include lost earnings and reasonable attorney' s fees—on a party or attorney who fails to comply.

    (2) *Command to Produce Materials or Permit Inspection.*

        (A) *Appearance Not Required.* A person commanded to produce documents, electronically stored information, or tangible things, or to permit the inspection of premises, need not appear in person at the place of production or inspection unless also commanded to appear for a deposition, hearing, or trial.

        (B) *Objections.* A person commanded to produce documents or tangible things or to permit inspection may serve on the party or attorney designated in the subpoena a written objection to inspecting, copying, testing or sampling any or all of the materials or to inspecting the premises—or to producing electronically stored information in the form or forms requested. The objection must be served before the earlier of the time specified for compliance or 14 days after the subpoena is served. If an objection is made, the following rules apply:

            (i) At any time, on notice to the commanded person, the serving party may move the court for the district where compliance is required for an order compelling production or inspection.

            (ii) These acts may be required only as directed in the order, and the order must protect a person who is neither a party nor a party's officer from significant expense resulting from compliance.

---

[2]From *Federal Rules of Civil Procedure, Title VI, Rule 45* (pp. 69–71), by the Committee on the Judiciary, House of Representatives, 2021 (https://www.uscourts.gov/sites/default/files/federal_rules_of_civil_procedure_dec_1_2021.pdf). In the public domain.

(3) *Quashing or Modifying a Subpoena.*

    (A) *When Required.* On timely motion, the court for the district where compliance is required must quash or modify a subpoena that:

        (i) fails to allow a reasonable time to comply;

        (ii) requires a person to comply beyond the geographical limits specified in Rule 45(c);

        (iii) requires disclosure of privileged or other protected matter, if no exception or waiver applies; or

        (iv) subjects a person to undue burden.

    (B) *When Permitted.* To protect a person subject to or affected by a subpoena, the court for the district where compliance is required may, on motion, quash or modify the subpoena if it requires:

        (i) disclosing a trade secret or other confidential research, development, or commercial information; or

        (ii) disclosing an unretained expert's opinion or information that does not describe specific occurrences in dispute and results from the expert's study that was not requested by a party.

    (C) *Specifying Conditions as an Alternative.* In the circumstances described in Rule 45(d)(3)(B), the court may, instead of quashing or modifying a subpoena, order appearance or production under specified conditions if the serving party:

        (iii) shows a substantial need for the testimony or material that cannot be otherwise met without undue hardship; and

        (iv) ensures that the subpoenaed person will be reasonably compensated.

(e) Duties in Responding to a Subpoena.

    (1) *Producing Documents or Electronically Stored Information.* These procedures apply to producing documents or electronically stored information:

    (A) *Documents.* A person responding to a subpoena to produce documents must produce them as they are kept in the ordinary course of business or must organize and label them to correspond to the categories in the demand.

    (B) *Form for Producing Electronically Stored Information Not Specified.* If a subpoena does not specify a form for producing electronically stored information, the person responding must produce it in a form or forms in which it is ordinarily maintained or in a reasonably usable form or forms.

(C) *Electronically Stored Information Produced in Only One Form.* The person responding need not produce the same electronically stored information in more than one form.

(D) *Inaccessible Electronically Stored Information.* The person responding need not provide discovery of electronically stored information from sources that the person identifies as not reasonably accessible because of undue burden or cost. On motion to compel discovery or for a protective order, the person responding must show that the information is not reasonably accessible because of undue burden or cost. If that showing is made, the court may nonetheless order discovery from such sources if the requesting party shows good cause, considering the limitations of Rule 26(b)(2)(C). The court may specify conditions for the discovery.

(2) *Claiming Privilege or Protection.*

(A) *Information Withheld.* A person withholding subpoenaed information under a claim that it is privileged or subject to protection as trial-preparation material must:

(i) expressly make the claim; and

(ii) describe the nature of the withheld documents, communications, or tangible things in a manner that, without revealing information itself privileged or protected, will enable the parties to assess the claim.

(B) *Information Produced.* If information produced in response to a subpoena is subject to a claim of privilege or of protection as trial-preparation material, the person making the claim may notify any party that received the information of the claim and the basis for it. After being notified, a party must promptly return, sequester, or destroy the specified information and any copies it has; must not use or disclose the information until the claim is resolved; must take reasonable steps to retrieve the information if the party disclosed it before being notified; and may promptly present the information under seal to the court for the district where compliance is required for a determination of the claim. The person who produced the information must preserve the information until the claim is resolved.

Appendix C

DISCLOSURE ISSUES

The following steps may be taken, as appropriate:

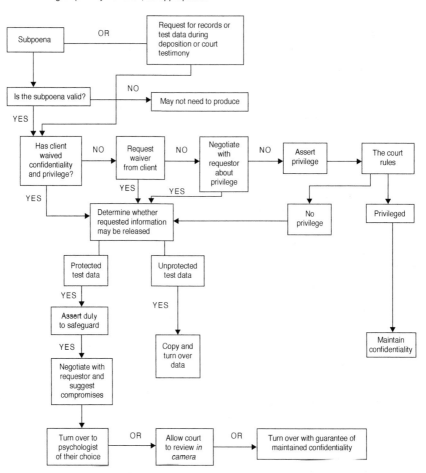

References

Abascal, A. M., Lillard, C. M., Law, K. B., & Jasinski, N. E. (2023). Curriculum Development for Competencies in Forensic Telemental Health Evaluations. *Journal of Technology in Behavioral Science, 9*, 14–19. https://doi.org/10.1007/s41347-023-00333-2

Adames, H. Y., & Chavez-Dueñas, N. Y. (2017). *Cultural foundations and interventions in Latino/a mental health: History, theory, and within group differences.* Routledge. https://doi.org/10.4324/9781315724058

Adames, H. Y., & Chavez-Dueñas, N. Y. (2021). Reclaiming all of me: The Racial Queer Identity Framework. In K. L. Nadal & M. Scharron del Rio (Eds.), *Queer psychology: Intersectional perspectives* (pp. 59–79). Springer. https://doi.org/10.1007/978-3-030-74146-4_4

Adames, H. Y., Chavez-Dueñas, N. Y., & Jernigan, M. M. (2021). The fallacy of a raceless Latinidad: Action guidelines for centering Blackness in Latinx psychology. *Journal of Latinx Psychology, 9*(1), 26–44. https://doi.org/10.1037/lat0000179

Adames, H. Y., Chavez-Dueñas, N. Y., & Jernigan, M. M. (2023). Dr. Janet E. Helms: Envisioning and creating a more humane psychological science, theory, and practice. *American Psychologist, 78*(4), 401–412. https://doi.org/10.1037/amp0001037

Adames, H. Y., Chavez-Dueñas, N. Y., Lewis, J. A., Neville, H. A., French, B. H., Chen, G. A., & Mosley, D. V. (2023). Radical healing in psychotherapy: Addressing the wounds of racism-related stress and trauma. *Psychotherapy, 60*(1), 39–50. https://doi.org/10.1037/pst0000435

Adames, H. Y., Chavez-Dueñas, N. Y., Sharma, S., & La Roche, M. J. (2018). Intersectionality in psychotherapy: The experiences of an AfroLatinx queer immigrant. *Psychotherapy, 55*(1), 73–79. https://doi.org/10.1037/pst0000152

Adames, H. Y., Chavez-Dueñas, N. Y., Vasquez, M. J. T., & Pope, K. S. (2023). *Succeeding as a therapist: How to create a thriving practice in a changing world.* American Psychological Association. https://doi.org/10.1037/0000321-000

Akamatsu, T. J. (1988). Intimate relationships with former clients: National survey of attitudes and behavior among practitioners. *Professional Psychology: Research and Practice, 19*(4), 454–458. https://doi.org/10.1037/0735-7028.19.4.454

Allen, J. G. (2022). *Trusting in psychotherapy.* American Psychiatric Association.

Allidina, S., & Cunningham, W. A. (2023). Motivated categories: Social structures shape the construction of social categories through attentional mechanisms. *Personality and Social Psychology Review, 27*(4), 393–413. https://doi.org/10.1177/10888683231172255

Alpert, J. L., & Steinberg, A. (2017). Sexual boundary violations: A century of violations and a time to analyze. *Psychoanalytic Psychology, 34*(2), 144–150. https://doi.org/10.1037/pap0000094

American Educational Research Association, American Psychological Association, & National Council on Measurement in Education. (2014). *Standards for educational and psychological testing.* American Educational Research Association.

American Psychiatric Association. (2022). *Diagnostic and statistical manual of mental disorders* (5th ed., text rev.). https://doi.org/10.1176/appi.books.9780890425787

American Psychological Association. (1975). Report of task force on sex bias and sex-role stereotyping in psychotherapeutic practice. *American Psychologist, 30*(12), 1169–1175. https://doi.org/10.1037/0003-066X.30.12.1169

American Psychological Association. (2012). Guidelines for psychological practice with lesbian, gay, and bisexual clients. *American Psychologist, 67*(1), 10–42. https://doi.org/10.1037/a0024659

American Psychological Association. (2013). Specialty guidelines for forensic psychology. *American Psychologist, 68*(1), 7–19. https://doi.org/10.1037/a0029889

American Psychological Association. (2015). Guidelines for psychological practice with transgender and gender nonconforming people. *American Psychologist, 70*(9), 832–864. https://doi.org/10.1037/a0039906

American Psychological Association. (2017). *Ethical principles of psychologists and code of conduct.* https://www.apa.org/ethics/code/ethics-code-2017.pdf

Archer, R. P., Wheeler, E. M. A., & Vauter, R. A. (2016). Empirically supported forensic assessment. *Clinical Psychology: Science and Practice, 23*(4), 348–364. https://doi.org/10.1111/cpsp.12171

Arkes, H. R., Faust, D., Guilmette, T. J., & Hart, K. (1988). Eliminating the hindsight bias. *Journal of Applied Psychology, 73*(2), 305–307. https://doi.org/10.1037/0021-9010.73.2.305

Bacon, F. (1955). *Selected writings of Francis Bacon.* Modern Library.

Bajt, T. R., & Pope, K. S. (1989). Therapist-patient sexual intimacy involving children and adolescents. *American Psychologist, 44*(2), 455. https://doi.org/10.1037/0003-066X.44.2.455

Baker, C. A., Baum, L. J., Francis, J. P., Shura, R. D., & Ord, A. S. (2023). Assessment of test bias on the MMPI-2-RF higher order and restructured clinical scales as a function of gender and race. *Professional Psychology: Research and Practice, 54*(4), 314–325. https://doi.org/10.1037/pro0000517

Barros, A. J. S., Rosa, R. G., & Eizirik, C. L. (2014). Countertransference reactions aroused by sex crimes in a forensic psychiatric environment. *International Journal of Forensic Mental Health, 13*(4), 363–368. https://doi.org/10.1080/14999013.2014.951106

Bártová, K., Androvičová, R., Krejčová, L., Weiss, P., & Klapilová, K. (2021). The prevalence of paraphilic interests in the Czech population: Preference, arousal, the use of pornography, fantasy, and behavior. *Journal of Sex Research, 58*(1), 86–96. https://doi.org/10.1080/00224499.2019.1707468

Batastini, A. B., Guyton, M. R., Bernhard, P. A., Folk, J. B., Knuth, S. B., Kohutis, E. A., Lugo, A., Stanfill, M. L., & Tussey, C. M. (2023). Recommendations for the use of telepsychology in psychology-law practice and research: A statement by American Psychology-Law Society (APA Division 41). *Psychology, Public Policy, and Law, 29*(3), 255–271. https://doi.org/10.1037/law0000394

Bates, C. M., & Brodsky, A. M. (1989). *Sex in the therapy hour: A case of professional incest.* Guilford Press.

Baylis, F. (1993). Therapist-patient sexual contact: A non consensual, inherently harmful activity. *Canadian Journal of Psychiatry, 38*(7), 502–506. https://doi.org/10.1177/070674379303800707

Ben-Ari, A., & Somer, E. (2004). The aftermath of therapist–client sex: Exploited women struggle with the consequences. *Clinical Psychology & Psychotherapy, 11*(2), 126–136. https://doi.org/10.1002/cpp.396

Ben-Porath, Y. S., Heilbrun, K., & Rizzo, M. (2022). Using the MMPI-3 in legal settings. *Journal of Personality Assessment, 104*(2), 162–178. https://doi.org/10.1080/00223891.2021.2006672

Bernsen, A., Tabachnick, B. G., & Pope, K. S. (1994). National survey of social workers' sexual attraction to their clients: Results, implications, and comparison to psychologists. *Ethics & Behavior, 4*(4), 369–388. https://doi.org/10.1207/s15327019eb0404_4

Blechner, M. (2021). Dissociation among psychoanalysts about sexual boundary violations. In C. Levin (Ed.), *Sexual boundary trouble in psychoanalysis* (pp 160–170). Routledge.

Bonham, V. L., Warshauer-Baker, E., & Collins, F. S. (2005). Race and ethnicity in the genome era: The complexity of the constructs. *American Psychologist, 60*(1), 9–15. https://doi.org/10.1037/0003-066X.60.1.9

Boone, K. B., Sweet, J. J., Byrd, D. A., Denney, R. L., Hanks, R. A., Kaufmann, P. M., Kirkwood, M. W., Larrabee, G. J., Marcopulos, B. A., Morgan, J. E., Paltzer, J. Y., Rivera Mindt, M., Schroeder, R. W., Sim, A. H., & Suhr, J. A. (2022). Official position of the American Academy of Clinical Neuropsychology on test security. *The Clinical Neuropsychologist, 36*(3), 523–545. https://doi.org/10.1080/13854046.2021.2022214

Borys, D. S., & Pope, K. S. (1989). Dual relationships between therapist and client: A national study of psychologists, psychiatrists, and social workers. *Professional Psychology: Research and Practice, 20*(5), 283–293. https://doi.org/10.1037/0735-7028.20.5.283

Bouhoutsos, J., Holroyd, J., Lerman, H., Forer, B. R., & Greenberg, M. (1983). Sexual intimacy between psychotherapists and patients. *Professional Psychology: Research and Practice, 14*(2), 185–196. https://doi.org/10.1037/0735-7028.14.2.185

Brabant, E., Falzeder, E., & Giampieri-Deutsch, P. (1993). *The correspondence of Sigmund Freud and Sándor Ferenczi* (P. T. Hoffer, Trans.; Vol. 1). Harvard University Press.

Brodsky, S. L. (2023). *Testifying in court: Guidelines and maxims for the expert witness* (3rd ed.). American Psychological Association. https://doi.org/10.1037/0000325-000

Brodsky, S. L., & Goldenson, J. (2022). Feedback in forensic mental health assessment. *Journal of Forensic Psychology Research and Practice, 24*(3), 359–371. https://doi.org/10.1080/24732850.2022.2124140

Brodsky, S. L., & Pope, K. S. (2023). Common flaws in forensic reports. *Professional Psychology: Research and Practice, 54*(6), 413–417. https://doi.org/10.1037/pro0000531

Brooks, S. (2010). Hypersexualization and the dark body: Race and inequality among Black and Latina women in the exotic dance industry. *Sexuality Research & Social Policy, 7*(2), 70–80. https://doi.org/10.1007/s13178-010-0010-5

Brown, L. S. (1988). Harmful effects of posttermination sexual and romantic relationships between therapists and their former clients. *Psychotherapy: Theory, Research, Practice, Training, 25*(2), 249–255. https://doi.org/10.1037/h0085339

Brown, R. (1958). *Words and things.* Free Press.

Brown, S., Bowen, E., & Prescott, D. (Eds.). (2017). *The forensic psychologist's report writing guide.* Taylor & Francis. https://doi.org/10.4324/9781315732152

Burgess, J. A. (1984). Principles and techniques of cross-examination. In B. G. Warschaw (Ed.), *The trial masters: A handbook of strategies and tactics that win cases* (pp. 249–255). Prentice-Hall.

Butcher, J. N., Graham, J. R., Ben-Porath, Y. S., Tellegen, A., Dahlstrom, W. G., & Kaemmer, B. (2001). *MMPI-2: Manual for administration and scoring* (Rev. ed.). University of Minnesota Press.

Butcher, J. N., Graham, J. R., Tellegen, A., & Kaemmer, B. (1989). *Manual for the restandardized Minnesota Multiphasic Personality Inventory: MMPI-2.* University of Minnesota Press.

Butler, S., & Zelen, S. L. (1977). Sexual intimacies between therapists and patients. *Psychotherapy: Theory, Research & Practice, 14*(2), 139–145. https://doi.org/10.1037/h0086521

Capawana, M. R. (2016). Intimate attractions and sexual misconduct in the therapeutic relationship: Implications for socially just practice. *Cogent Psychology*,
3(1), Article 1194176. https://doi.org/10.1080/23311908.2016.1194176

Carey, B. (2011, November 2). Fraud case seen as a red flag for psychology
research. *The New York Times*. https://www.nytimes.com/2011/11/03/health/
research/noted-dutch-psychologist-stapel-accused-of-research-fraud.html

Carpenter, M. (2018). Intersex variations, human rights, and the international
classification of diseases. *Health and Human Rights*, *20*(2), 205–214.

Carter, R. T., & Pieterse, A. L. (2005). Race: A social and psychological analysis
of the term and its meaning. In R. T. Carter (Ed.), *Handbook of racial-cultural
psychology and counseling* (pp. 41–63). Wiley.

Chandrashekar, S. P., Yeung, S. K., Yau, K. C., Cheung, C. Y., Agarwal, T. K., Wong,
C. Y. J., Pillai, T., Thirlwell, T. N., Leung, W. N., Tse, C., Li, Y. T., Cheng, B. L.,
Chan, H. Y. C., & Feldman, G. (2021). Agency and self-other asymmetries in
perceived bias and shortcomings: Replications of the Bias Blind Spot and link
to free will beliefs. *Judgment and Decision Making*, *16*(6), 1392–1412. https://
doi.org/10.1017/S1930297500008470

Chavez-Dueñas, N. Y., & Adames, H. Y. (2022). Parenting while undocumented:
An intersectional socialization approach. *Current Opinion in Psychology*, *47*,
101441. https://doi.org/10.1016/j.copsyc.2022.101441

Chavez-Dueñas, N. Y., Adames, H. Y., Perez-Chavez, J. G., & Salas, S. P. (2019).
Healing ethno-racial trauma in Latinx immigrant communities: Cultivating
hope, resistance, and action. *American Psychologist*, *74*(1), 49–62. https://
doi.org/10.1037/amp0000289

Chesler, P. (1971). Patient and patriarch: Women in the psychotherapeutic relationship. In V. Gornick & B. K. Moran (Eds.), *Woman in sexist society: Studies in
power and powerlessness* (pp. 362–392). Basic Books.

Chesler, P. (1972). *Women and madness*. Palgrave Macmillan.

Combahee River Collective. (1995). Combahee River Collective statement. In
B. Guy-Sheftall (Ed.), *Words of fire: An anthology of African American feminist
thought* (pp. 232–240). New Press.

Committee on Legal Issues, American Psychological Association. (2016). Strategies for private practitioners coping with subpoenas or compelled testimony for client/patient records or test data or test materials. *Professional
Psychology: Research and Practice*, *47*(1), 1–11. https://doi.org/10.1037/
pro0000063

Contreras, J. M., Banaji, M. R., & Mitchell, J. P. (2013). Multivoxel patterns
in fusiform face area differentiate faces by sex and race. *PLOS ONE*, *8*(7),
Article e69684. https://doi.org/10.1371/journal.pone.0069684

Courtois, C. A. (2017). Colleague betrayal: Countertrauma manifestation? In
R. B. Gartner (Ed.), *Trauma and countertrauma, resilience and counterresilience:
Insights from psychoanalysts and trauma experts* (pp. 251–281). Routledge/
Taylor & Francis Group.

Crenshaw, K. W. (1991). Mapping the margins: Intersectionality, identity politics, and violence against women of color. *Stanford Law Review, 43*(6), 1241–1299. https://doi.org/10.2307/1229039

Dahlberg, C. C. (1970). Sexual contact between patient and therapist. *Contemporary Psychoanalysis, 6*(2), 107–124. https://doi.org/10.1080/00107530.1970.10745180

Davidson, V. (1977). Psychiatry's problem with no name: Therapist–patient sex. *The American Journal of Psychoanalysis, 37*(1), 43–50. https://doi.org/10.1007/BF01252822

Davis, R. L., & Mitchell, M. (Eds.). (2021). *Heterosexual histories*. NYU Press.

DeMier, R. L., & Otto, R. K. (2017). Forensic report writing: Principles and challenges. In R. Roesch & A. N. Cook (Eds.), *Handbook of forensic mental health services* (pp. 216–234). Routledge. https://doi.org/10.4324/9781315627823-8

Diamond, L. M. (2007). A dynamical systems approach to the development and expression of female same-sex sexuality. *Perspectives on Psychological Science, 2*(2), 142–161. https://doi.org/10.1111/j.1745-6916.2007.00034.x

dickey, l. m. (2023). Exploring sex and gender diversity. In A. M. Schubert & M. Pope (Eds.), *Handbook for human sexuality counseling: A sex positive approach* (pp. 159–172). American Counseling Association.

Dixon, J. N., Caddell, T. M., Alexander, A. A., Burchett, D., Anderson, J. L., Marek, R. J., & Glassmire, D. M. (2023). Adapting assessment processes to consider cultural mistrust in forensic practices: An example with the MMPI instruments. *Law and Human Behavior, 47*(1), 292–306. https://doi.org/10.1037/lhb0000504

Dr. K v. State Board of Physician Quality Assurance, 98 Md. App. 103, 632, A.2d 453 (1993).

Dror, I. E., Kukucka, J., Kassin, S. M., & Zapf, P. A. (2018). When expert decision making goes wrong: Consensus, bias, the role of experts, and accuracy. *Journal of Applied Research in Memory and Cognition, 7*(1), 162–163. https://doi.org/10.1016/j.jarmac.2018.01.007

Durré, L. (1980). Comparing romantic and therapeutic relationships. In K. S. Pope (Ed.), *On love and loving: Psychological perspectives on the nature and experience of romantic love* (pp. 228–243). Jossey-Bass.

Ehrlinger, J., Gilovich, T., & Ross, L. (2005). Peering into the bias blind spot: People's assessments of bias in themselves and others. *Personality and Social Psychology Bulletin, 31*(5), 680–692. https://doi.org/10.1177/0146167204271570

Erdberg, S. P. (1970). MMPI differences associated with sex, race, and residence in a Southern sample. *Dissertation Abstracts International: Section B. Sciences and Engineering, 30*(11-B), 5236.

Erdberg, S. P. (1988, August 12–16). *How clinicians can achieve competence in testing procedures* [Paper presentation]. American Psychological Association 96th Annual Convention, Atlanta, GA, United States.

Essed, P. (1991). *Understanding everyday racism: An interdisciplinary theory*. Sage. https://doi.org/10.4135/9781483345239

Falzeder, E., Brabant, E., & Giampieri-Deutsch, P. (Eds.). (1996). *The correspondence of Sigmund Freud and Sándor Ferenczi* (P. T. Hoffer, Trans.; Vol. 2). Harvard University Press.

Falzeder, E., Brabant, E., & Giampieri-Deutsch, P. (Eds.). (2000). *The correspondence of Sigmund Freud and Sándor Ferenczi* (P. T. Hoffer, Trans.; Vol. 3). Harvard University Press.

Faschingbauer, T. R. (1979). The future of the MMPI. In C. S. Newmark (Ed.), *MMPI: Clinical and research trends* (pp. 373–398). Praeger.

Federal Rules of Civil Procedure, Title VI, Rule 45(c), 28 U.S.C. (2014). https://uscode.house.gov/view.xhtml?path=/prelim@title28/title28a/node88/node143&edition=prelim

Federal Rules of Civil Procedure, Title VI, Rule 45 (2021). https://www.uscourts.gov/sites/default/files/federal_rules_of_civil_procedure_dec_1_2021.pdf

Feldman-Summers, S., & Jones, G. (1984). Psychological impacts of sexual contact between therapists or other health care practitioners and their clients. *Journal of Consulting and Clinical Psychology, 52*(6), 1054–1061. https://doi.org/10.1037/0022-006X.52.6.1054

Finkelhor, D. (1984). *Child sexual abuse: New theory and research*. Free Press.

Fischhoff, B. (1975). Hindsight is not equal to foresight: The effect of outcome knowledge on judgment under uncertainty. *Journal of Experimental Psychology: Human Perception and Performance, 1*(3), 288–299. https://doi.org/10.1037/0096-1523.1.3.288

Fischhoff, B., & Beyth, R. (1975). I knew it would happen: Remembered probabilities of once-future things. *Organizational Behavior and Human Performance, 13*(1), 1–16. https://doi.org/10.1016/0030-5073(75)90002-1

Folman, R. Z. (1991). Therapist-patient sex: Attraction and boundary problems. *Psychotherapy: Theory, Research, Practice, Training, 28*(1), 168–173. https://doi.org/10.1037/0033-3204.28.1.168

Forer, B. R. (1980, February). *The therapeutic relationship: 1968* [Paper presentation]. California Psychological Association, Pasadena, CA, United States.

Freeman, L., & Roy, J. (1976). *Betrayal*. Stein & Day.

Frennette, L. (1991). *Abus de pouvoir* [Abuse of power]. Les Presses d'Amérique.

Freud, S. (1915). Observations on transference-love (Further recommendations on the technique of psycho-analysis III). In J. Strachey (Ed. & Trans.), *The standard edition of the complete psychological works of Sigmund Freud* (Vol. 12, pp. 157–171). Hogarth Press. (Original work published 1912)

Freud, S. (1924). The future prospects of psycho-analytic therapy. In J. Riviere (Trans.), *The collected papers of Sigmund Freud* (Vol. 2, pp. 285–296). Hogarth Press. (Original work published 1910)

Gabbard, G. O. (1991). Psychodynamics of sexual boundary violations. *Psychiatric Annals, 21*(11), 651–655. https://doi.org/10.3928/0048-5713-19911101-06

Garnets, L. D., & Kimmel, D. C. (Eds.). (2003). *Psychological perspectives on lesbian, gay, and bisexual experiences* (2nd ed.). Columbia University Press.

Gartrell, N., Herman, J., Olarte, S., Feldstein, M., & Localio, R. (1986). Psychiatrist-patient sexual contact: Results of a national survey. I: Prevalence. *The American Journal of Psychiatry, 143*(9), 1126–1131. https://doi.org/10.1176/ajp.143.9.1126

Gavett, B. E., Lynch, J. K., & McCaffrey, R. J. (2005). Third party observers: The effect size is greater than you might think. *Journal of Forensic Neuropsychology, 4*(2), 49–64. https://doi.org/10.1300/J151v04n02_05

Gechtman, L. (1989). Sexual contact between social workers and their clients. In G. O. Gabbard (Ed.), *Sexual exploitation in professional relationships* (pp. 27–38). American Psychiatric Press.

Gechtman, L., & Bouhoutsos, J. (1985, October). *Sexual intimacy between social workers and clients* [Paper presentation]. Society for Clinical Social Workers Annual Meeting, Universal City, CA, United States.

Gibson, W. T., & Pope, K. S. (1993). The ethics of counseling: A national survey of certified counselors. *Journal of Counseling & Development, 71*(3), 330–336. https://doi.org/10.1002/j.1556-6676.1993.tb02222.x

Gilovich, T., Griffin, D., & Kahneman, D. (Eds.). (2002). *Heuristics and biases: The psychology of intuitive judgment.* Cambridge University Press. https://doi.org/10.1017/CBO9780511808098

Glen, T., Barisa, M., Ready, R., Peck, E., & Spencer, T. R. (2021). Update on third party observers in neuropsychological evaluation: An Interorganizational position paper. *The Clinical Neuropsychologist, 35*(6), 1107–1116. https://doi.org/10.1080/13854046.2021.1901992

Goldenson, J., Brodsky, S. L., & Perlin, M. L. (2022). Trauma-informed forensic mental health assessment: Practical implications, ethical tensions, and alignment with therapeutic jurisprudence principles. *Psychology, Public Policy, and Law, 28*(2), 226–239. https://doi.org/10.1037/law0000339

Goldenson, J., & Gutheil, T. (2023). Forensic mental health evaluators' unprocessed emotions as an often-overlooked form of bias. *The Journal of the American Academy of Psychiatry and the Law, 51*(4), 551–557.

Goldenson, J., & Josefowitz, N. (2021). Remote forensic psychological assessment in civil cases: Considerations for experts assessing harms from early life abuse. *Psychological Injury and Law, 14*(2), 89–103. https://doi.org/10.1007/s12207-021-09404-2

Goldenson, J., Nijdam-Jones, A., Druhn, N., Hill, D., Coupland, S., & Roesch, R. (2023). The practice of clinical forensic psychology in Canada: Current landscape and future directions. *Canadian Psychology/Psychologie canadienne, 64*(4), 306–312. https://doi.org/10.1037/cap0000354

Goldyne, A. J. (2007). Minimizing the influence of unconscious bias in evaluations: A practical guide. *Journal of the American Academy of Psychiatry and the Law, 35*(1), 60–66.

Gómez, J. M., Noll, L. K., Adams-Clark, A. A., & Courtois, C. A. (2021). When colleagues betray: The harm of sexual boundary violations in psychotherapy extends beyond the victim. In A. (L.) Steinberg, J. L. Alpert, & C. A. Courtois (Eds.), *Sexual boundary violations in psychotherapy: Facing therapist indiscretions, transgressions, and misconduct* (pp. 297–315). American Psychological Association. https://doi.org/10.1037/0000247-017

Greenberg, S. A., & Shuman, D. W. (2007). When worlds collide: Therapeutic and forensic roles. *Professional Psychology: Research and Practice, 38*(2), 129–132. https://doi.org/10.1037/0735-7028.38.2.129

Guilbault, R. L., Bryant, F. B., Brockway, J. H., & Posavac, E. J. (2004). A meta-analysis of research on hindsight bias. *Basic and Applied Social Psychology, 26*(2–3), 103–117. https://doi.org/10.1080/01973533.2004.9646399

Gutheil, T. G., & Brodsky, A. (2008). *Preventing boundary violations in clinical practice.* Guilford Press.

Gutheil, T. G., & Drogin, E. Y. (2013). *The mental health professional in court: A survival guide.* American Psychiatric Publishing.

Gutheil, T. G., & Gabbard, G. O. (1992). Obstacles to the dynamic understanding of therapist-patient sexual relations. *American Journal of Psychotherapy, 46*(4), 515–525. https://doi.org/10.1176/appi.psychotherapy.1992.46.4.515

Gynther, M. D., Fowler, R. D., & Erdberg, P. (1971). False positives galore: The application of standard MMPI criteria to a rural, isolated, Negro sample. *Journal of Clinical Psychology, 27*(2), 234–237. https://doi.org/10.1002/1097-4679(197104)27:2<234::AID-JCLP2270270225>3.0.CO;2-2

Hale, N. G. (Ed.). (1971). *James Jackson Putnam and psychoanalysis: Letters between Putnam and Sigmund Freud, Ernest Jones, William James, Sandor Ferenczi, and Morton Prince, 1877–1917.* Harvard University Press.

Hare-Mustin, R. T. (1974). Ethical considerations in the use of sexual contact in psychotherapy. *Psychotherapy: Theory, Research, & Practice, 11*(4), 308–310. https://doi.org/10.1037/h0086370

Harro, B. (2000). The cycle of socialization. In M. Adams, W. J. Blumenfeld, R. Castaneda, H. W. Hackman, M. L. Peters, & X. Zuniga (Eds.), *Readings for diversity and social justice* (pp. 15–21). Routledge.

Hathaway, S. R., & McKinley, J. C. (1943). *MMPI: Manual for administration and scoring.* University of Minnesota.

Health Insurance Portability and Accountability Act of 1996, Pub. L. No. 104–191, 110 Stat. 1936.

Helms, J. E. (1992). Why is there no study of cultural equivalence in standardized cognitive ability testing? *American Psychologist, 47*(9), 1083–1101. https://doi.org/10.1037/0003-066X.47.9.1083

Helms, J. E. (2008). *A race is a nice thing to have: A guide to being a White person or understanding the White persons in your life* (2nd ed.). Alexander Street Press.

Helms, J. E. (2015). An examination of the evidence in culturally adapted evidence-based or empirically supported interventions. *Transcultural Psychiatry, 52*(2), 174–197. https://doi.org/10.1177/1363461514563642

Helms, J. E., & Cook, D. A. (1999). *Using race and culture in counseling and psychotherapy: Theory and process*. Allyn & Bacon.

Helms, J. E., Jernigan, M., & Mascher, J. (2005). The meaning of race in psychology and how to change it: A methodological perspective. *American Psychologist, 60*(1), 27–36. https://doi.org/10.1037/0003-066X.60.1.27

Henley, N. M. (1971, September 3–7). *The politics of touch* [Paper presentation]. American Psychological Association 79th Annual Convention, Washington, DC, United States.

Herman, J. L. (2023). *Truth and repair: How trauma survivors envision justice*. Basic Books.

Herman, J. L., Gartrell, N., Olarte, S., Feldstein, M., & Localio, R. (1987). Psychiatrist-patient sexual contact: Results of a national survey, II: Psychiatrists' attitudes. *The American Journal of Psychiatry, 144*(2), 164–169. https://doi.org/10.1176/ajp.144.2.164

Holroyd, J. C., & Brodsky, A. M. (1977). Psychologists' attitudes and practices regarding erotic and nonerotic physical contact with patients. *American Psychologist, 32*(10), 843–849. https://doi.org/10.1037/0003-066X.32.10.843

Holt, R. (1964). Imagery: The return of the ostracized. *American Psychologist, 19*(4), 254–264. https://doi.org/10.1037/h0046316

Hornstein, G. A. (2000). *To redeem one person is to redeem the world: The life of Frieda Fromm-Reichmann*. Other Press.

Howe, L. L., & McCaffrey, R. J. (2010). Third party observation during neuropsychological evaluation: An update on the literature, practical advice for practitioners, and future directions. *The Clinical Neuropsychologist, 24*(3), 518–537. https://doi.org/10.1080/13854041003775347

Janoff-Bulman, R., Timko, C., & Carli, L. L. (1985). Cognitive biases in blaming the victim. *Journal of Experimental Social Psychology, 21*(2), 161–177. https://doi.org/10.1016/0022-1031(85)90013-7

Jehu, D. (1994). *Patients as victims: Sexual abuse in psychotherapy and counselling*. Wiley.

Jones, C. P. (2000). Levels of racism: A theoretic framework and a gardener's tale. *American Journal of Public Health, 90*(8), 1212–1215. https://doi.org/10.2105/AJPH.90.8.1212

Jones, J. M. (1972). *Prejudice and racism*. Addison-Wesley.

Joyal, C. (2017). Sexual fantasy. In T. Shackelford & V. Weekes-Shackelford (Eds.), *Encyclopedia of evolutionary psychological science* (pp. 1–3). Springer. https://doi.org/10.1007/978-3-319-16999-6_3363-1

Joyal, C. C., & Carpentier, J. (2017). The prevalence of paraphilic interests and behaviors in the general population: A provincial survey. *Journal of Sex Research, 54*(2), 161–171. https://doi.org/10.1080/00224499.2016.1139034

Joyal, C. C., Cossette, A., & Lapierre, V. (2015). What exactly is an unusual sexual fantasy? *Journal of Sexual Medicine, 12*(2), 328–340. https://doi.org/10.1111/jsm.12734

Kahneman, D. (2011). *Thinking, fast and slow*. Farrar, Straus & Giroux.

Kahneman, D., Sibony, O., & Sunstein, C. R. (2021). *Noise: A flaw in human judgment.* Little, Brown Spark.

Karson, M., & Nadkarni, L. (2013). *Principles of forensic report writing.* American Psychological Association. https://doi.org/10.1037/14182-000

Katz, J. N. (1995). *The invention of heterosexuality.* University of Chicago Press.

King, D. E. (2022). The inclusion of sex and gender beyond the binary in toxicology. *Frontiers in Toxicology, 4,* Article 929219. https://doi.org/10.3389/ftox.2022.929219

Kinsey, A. C., Pomeroy, W. B., Martin, C. E., & Gebhard, P. H. (1953). *Sexual behavior in the human female.* Saunders.

Koocher, G. P. (2006). Foreword to the second edition: Things my teachers never mentioned. In K. S. Pope, J. L. Sonne, & B. G. Greene, *What therapists don't talk about and why: Understanding taboos that hurt us and our clients* (pp. xxi–xxiv). American Psychological Association. https://doi.org/10.1037/11413-000

Koriat, A., Lichtenstein, S., & Fischhoff, B. (1980). Reasons for confidence. *Journal of Experimental Psychology: Human Learning and Memory, 6*(2), 107–118. https://doi.org/10.1037/0278-7393.6.2.107

Kukucka, J., Kassin, S. M., Zapf, P. A., & Dror, I. E. (2017). Cognitive bias and blindness: A global survey of forensic science examiners. *Journal of Applied Research in Memory and Cognition, 6*(4), 452–459. https://doi.org/10.1016/j.jarmac.2017.09.001

Laqueur, T. (1992). *Making sex: Body and gender from the Greeks to Freud.* Harvard University Press.

Lawson, A. K., Fitzgerald, L. F., & Collinsworth, L. L. (2022). Computerized test interpretation of the MMPI-2 in the forensic context: A time to use your head and not the formula? *Psychological Injury and Law, 16*(2), 199–212. https://doi.org/10.1007/s12207-022-09465-x

Lehmiller, J. J. (2018). *Tell me what you want: The science of sexual desire and how it can help you improve your sex life.* Da Capo Lifelong Books.

Lehmiller, J. J., & Gormezano, A. M. (2023). Sexual fantasy research: A contemporary review. *Current Opinion in Psychology, 49,* Article 101496. https://doi.org/10.1016/j.copsyc.2022.101496

Leitenberg, H., & Henning, K. (1995). Sexual fantasy. *Psychological Bulletin, 117*(3), 469–496. https://doi.org/10.1037/0033-2909.117.3.469

Levin, C. (2021). *Social aspects of sexual boundary trouble in psychoanalysis.* Taylor & Francis.

Lewandowski, A., Baker, W. J., Sewick, B., Knippa, J., Axelrod, B., & McCaffrey, R. J. (2016). Policy statement of the American Board of Professional Neuropsychology regarding third party observation and the recording of psychological test administration in neuropsychological evaluations [Editorial]. *Applied Neuropsychology: Adult, 23*(6), 391–398. https://doi.org/10.1080/23279095.2016.1176366

Lewis, J. A., Mendenhall, R., Harwood, S. A., & Browne Huntt, M. (2016). "Ain't I a woman?": Perceived gendered racial microaggressions experienced by Black women. *The Counseling Psychologist, 44*(5), 758–780. https://doi.org/10.1177/0011000016641193

Lewis, J. A., & Neville, H. A. (2015). Construction and initial validation of the Gendered Racial Microaggressions Scale for Black women. *Journal of Counseling Psychology, 62*(2), 289–302. https://doi.org/10.1037/cou0000062

Lindley, L. M., Anzani, A., Prunas, A., & Galupo, M. P. (2020). Sexual fantasy across gender identity: A qualitative investigation of differences between cisgender and non-binary people's imagery. *Sexual and Relationship Therapy, 37*(2), 157–178. https://doi.org/10.1080/14681994.2020.1716966

Martin, G. M., & Beaulieu, I. (2023). Sexual misconduct: What does a 20-year review of cases in Quebec reveal about the characteristics of professionals, victims, and the disciplinary process? *Sexual Abuse.* Advance online publication. https://doi.org/10.1177/10790632231170818

Masters, W. H., & Johnson, V. E. (1966). *Human sexual response.* Little, Brown.

Masters, W. H., & Johnson, V. E. (1970). *Human sexual inadequacy.* Bantam Books.

Masters, W. H., & Johnson, V. E. (1976). Principles of the new sex therapy. *The American Journal of Psychiatry, 133*(5), 548–554. https://doi.org/10.1176/ajp.133.5.548

McAuliff, B. D., & Arter, J. L. (2016). Adversarial allegiance: The devil is in the evidence details, not just on the witness stand. *Law and Human Behavior, 40*(5), 524–535. https://doi.org/10.1037/lhb0000198

Morandini, J. S., Dacosta, L., & Dar-Nimrod, I. (2021). Exposure to continuous or fluid theories of sexual orientation leads some heterosexuals to embrace less-exclusive heterosexual orientations. *Scientific Reports, 11*(1), Article 16546. https://doi.org/10.1038/s41598-021-94479-9

Mukkamala, S., & Suyemoto, K. L. (2018). Racialized sexism/sexualized racism: A multimethod study of intersectional experiences of discrimination for Asian American women. *Asian American Journal of Psychology, 9*(1), 32–46. https://doi.org/10.1037/aap0000104

Murrie, D. C., & Boccaccini, M. T. (2015). Adversarial allegiance among expert witnesses. *Annual Review of Law and Social Science, 11*(1), 37–55. https://doi.org/10.1146/annurev-lawsocsci-120814-121714

Murrie, D. C., Boccaccini, M. T., Guarnera, L. A., & Rufino, K. A. (2013). Are forensic experts biased by the side that retained them? *Psychological Science, 24*(10), 1889–1897. https://doi.org/10.1177/0956797613481812

Murrie, D. C., Boccaccini, M. T., Turner, D. B., Meeks, M., Woods, C., & Tussey, C. (2009). Rater (dis)agreement on risk assessment measures in sexually violent predator proceedings: Evidence of adversarial allegiance in forensic evaluation? *Psychology, Public Policy, and Law, 15*(1), 19–53. https://doi.org/10.1037/a0014897

Nachmani, I., & Somer, E. (2007). Women sexually victimized in psychotherapy speak out: The dynamics and outcome of therapist–client sex. *Women & Therapy, 30*(1–2), 1–17. https://doi.org/10.1300/J015v30n01_01

Nakamura, N., Dispenza, F., Abreu, R. L., Ollen, E. W., Pantalone, D. W., Canillas, G., Gormley, B., & Vencill, J. A. (2022). The APA Guidelines for Psychological Practice With Sexual Minority Persons: An executive summary of the 2021 revision. *American Psychologist, 77*(8), 953–962. https://doi.org/10.1037/amp0000939

National Academies of Sciences, Engineering, and Medicine. (2022). *Measuring sex, gender identity, and sexual orientation.* https://doi.org/10.17226/26424

Neal, T. M. S., & Brodsky, S. L. (2016). Forensic psychologists' perceptions of bias and potential correction strategies in forensic mental health evaluations. *Psychology, Public Policy, and Law, 22*(1), 58–76. https://doi.org/10.1037/law0000077

Neal, T. M. S., & Line, E. N. (2022, July 6). Income, demographics, and life experiences of clinical-forensic psychologists in the United States. *Frontiers in Psychology, 13,* Article 910672. https://doi.org/10.3389/fpsyg.2022.910672

Neblett, E. W., Jr., White, R. L., Ford, K. R., Philip, C. L., Nguyen, H. X., & Sellers, R. M. (2008). Patterns of racial socialization and psychological adjustment: Can parental communications about race reduce the impact of racial discrimination? *Journal of Research on Adolescence, 18*(3), 477–515. https://doi.org/10.1111/j.1532-7795.2008.00568.x

Neisser, U. (1967). *Cognitive psychology.* Appleton-Century-Crofts.

Neville, H. A., Awad, G. H., Brooks, J. E., Flores, M. P., & Bluemel, J. (2013). Color-blind racial ideology: Theory, training, and measurement implications in psychology. *American Psychologist, 68*(6), 455–466. https://doi.org/10.1037/a0033282

Neville, H. A., Lilly, R. L., Duran, G., Lee, R. M., & Browne, L. (2000). Construction and initial validation of the Color-Blind Racial Attitudes Scale (CoBRAS). *Journal of Counseling Psychology, 47*(1), 59–70. https://doi.org/10.1037/0022-0167.47.1.59

Noël, B., & Watterson, K. (1992). *You must be dreaming.* Poseidon Press.

Nugent, C. D. (1994). Blaming the victims: Silencing women sexually exploited by psychotherapists. *Journal of Mind and Behavior, 15*(1–2), 113–138.

Otto, R. K. (1989). Bias and expert testimony of mental health professionals in adversarial proceedings: A preliminary investigation. *Behavioral Sciences & the Law, 7*(2), 267–273. https://doi.org/10.1002/bsl.2370070210

Otto, R. K., DeMier, R., & Boccaccini, M. (2014). *Forensic reports and testimony: A guide to effective communication for psychologists and psychiatrists.* Wiley.

Pace, E. (1994, November 15). Jules Masserman, 89, leader of psychiatric group, is dead. *The New York Times.* https://www.nytimes.com/1994/11/15/obituaries/jules-masserman-89-leader-of-psychiatric-group-is-dead.html

Paivio, A. (1971). *Imagery and verbal processes.* Holt, Rinehart, & Winston.

Palfreman, C. (2023). The use of telemedicine in forensic psychiatry—A quick scoping review of literature from the time of the COVID-19 pandemic. *Journal of Forensic Psychiatry & Psychology, 34*(1), 81–93. https://doi.org/10.1080/14789949.2023.2174161

Penfold, P. S. (1987). Sexual abuse between therapist and woman patient. *Canadian Woman Studies/les cahiers de la femme, 8*(4), 29–31.

Penfold, P. S. (1992). Sexual abuse by therapists: Maintaining the conspiracy of silence. *Canadian Journal of Community Mental Health, 11*(1), 5–15. https://doi.org/10.7870/cjcmh-1992-0001

Penfold, P. S. (1998). *Sexual abuse by health professionals: A personal search for meaning and healing.* University of Toronto Press. https://doi.org/10.3138/9781442679832

Penfold, P. S. (1999). Why did you keep going for so long? Issues for survivors of long-term, sexually abusive "helping" relationships. *Journal of Sex Education & Therapy, 24*(4), 244–251. https://doi.org/10.1080/01614576.1999.11074312

Peplau, L. A., & Garnets, L. D. (2000). A new paradigm for understanding women's sexuality and sexual orientation. *Journal of Social Issues, 56*(2), 330–350. https://doi.org/10.1111/0022-4537.00169

Perillo, J. T., Perillo, A. D., Despodova, N. M., & Kovera, M. B. (2021). Testing the waters: An investigation of the impact of hot tubbing on experts from referral through testimony. *Law and Human Behavior, 45*(3), 229–242. https://doi.org/10.1037/lhb0000446

Pismenny, A. (2023). Pansexuality: A closer look at sexual orientation. *Philosophies, 8*(4), Article 60. https://doi.org/10.3390/philosophies8040060

Plasil, E. (1985). *Therapist.* St. Martin's/Marek.

Pope, K. S. (1988). How clients are harmed by sexual contact with mental health professionals: The syndrome and its prevalence. *Journal of Counseling & Development, 67*(4), 222–226. https://doi.org/10.1002/j.1556-6676.1988.tb02587.x

Pope, K. S. (1990a). Therapist-patient sex as sex abuse: Six scientific, professional, and practical dilemmas in addressing victimization and rehabilitation. *Professional Psychology: Research and Practice, 21*(4), 227–239. https://doi.org/10.1037/0735-7028.21.4.227

Pope, K. S. (1990b). Therapist-patient sexual involvement: A review of the research. *Clinical Psychology Review, 10*(4), 477–490. https://doi.org/10.1016/0272-7358(90)90049-G

Pope, K. S. (1992). Responsibilities in providing psychological test feedback to clients. *Psychological Assessment, 4*(3), 268–271. https://doi.org/10.1037/1040-3590.4.3.268

Pope, K. S. (1993). Licensing disciplinary actions for psychologists who have been sexually involved with a client: Some information about offenders. *Professional Psychology: Research and Practice, 24*(3), 374–377. https://doi.org/10.1037/0735-7028.24.3.374

Pope, K. S. (1994). *Sexual involvement with therapists: Patient assessment, subsequent therapy, forensics.* American Psychological Association. https://doi.org/10.1037/10154-000

Pope, K. S., & Bouhoutsos, J. C. (1986). *Sexual intimacy between therapists and patients.* Praeger.

Pope, K. S., Butcher, J. N., & Seelen, J. (2006). *The MMPI, MMPI-2, & MMPI-A in court: A practical guide for expert witnesses and attorneys* (3rd ed.). American Psychological Association. https://doi.org/10.1037/11437-000

Pope, K. S., Chavez-Dueñas, N. Y., Adames, H. Y., Sonne, J. L., & Greene, B. A. (2023). *Speaking the unspoken: Breaking the silence, myths, and taboos that hurt therapists and patients.* American Psychological Association. https://doi.org/10.1037/0000350-000

Pope, K. S., & Feldman-Summers, S. (1992). National survey of psychologists' sexual and physical abuse history and their evaluation of training and competence in these areas. *Professional Psychology: Research and Practice, 23*(5), 353–361. https://doi.org/10.1037/0735-7028.23.5.353

Pope, K. S., Keith-Spiegel, P., & Tabachnick, B. G. (1986). Sexual attraction to clients: The human therapist and the (sometimes) inhuman training system. *American Psychologist, 41*(2), 147–158. https://doi.org/10.1037/0003-066X.41.2.147

Pope, K. S., Levenson, H., & Schover, L. R. (1979). Sexual intimacy in psychology training: Results and implications of a national survey. *American Psychologist, 34*(8), 682–689. https://doi.org/10.1037/0003-066X.34.8.682

Pope, K. S., & Singer, J. L. (Eds.). (1978). *The stream of consciousness: Scientific investigations into the flow of human experience.* Plenum. https://doi.org/10.1007/978-1-4684-2466-9

Pope, K. S., Singer, J. L., & Rosenberg, L. C. (1984). Sex, fantasy and imagination: Scientific research and clinical applications. In A. Sheikh (Ed.), *Imagination and healing* (pp. 197–209). Baywood.

Pope, K. S., Tabachnick, B. G., & Keith-Spiegel, P. (1987). Ethics of practice: The beliefs and behaviors of psychologists as therapists. *American Psychologist, 42*(11), 993–1006. https://doi.org/10.1037/0003-066X.42.11.993

Pope, K. S., Vasquez, M. J. T., Chavez-Dueñas, N. Y., & Adames, H. Y. (2021). *Ethics in psychotherapy and counseling: A practical guide* (6th ed.). Wiley. https://doi.org/10.1002/9781394259038

Pope, K. S., & Vetter, V. A. (1991). Prior therapist-patient sexual involvement among patients seen by psychologists. *Psychotherapy: Theory, Research, Practice, Training, 28*(3), 429–438. https://doi.org/10.1037/0033-3204.28.3.429

Pronin, E., & Hazel, L. (2023). Humans' bias blind spot and its societal significance. *Current Directions in Psychological Science, 32*(5), 402–409. https://doi.org/10.1177/09637214231178745

Pronin, E., Lin, D. Y., & Ross, L. (2002). The bias blind spot: Perceptions of bias in self versus others. *Personality and Social Psychology Bulletin, 28*(3), 369–381. https://doi.org/10.1177/0146167202286008

Psychotherapy Notes, 45 C.F.R. § 164.501 (2023). https://www.govinfo.gov/content/pkg/CFR-2023-title45-vol2/pdf/CFR-2023-title45-vol2-sec164-501.pdf

Rather, D. (Self-Correspondent). (1978, September 10). 50 Minutes (Season 10, Episode 53) [TV series episode]. In S. Glauber, M. Goldin, & J. Wershba (Producers). *60 Minutes*. CBS Television.

Ratkalkar, M., Jackson, C., & Heilbrun, K. (2023). Race-informed forensic mental health assessment: A principles-based analysis. *International Journal of Forensic Mental Health, 22*(4), 314–325. https://doi.org/10.1080/14999013.2023.2178556

Reeder, D. J., & Schatte, D. J. (2011). Managing negative reactions in forensic trainees. *The Journal of the American Academy of Psychiatry and the Law, 39*(2), 217–221.

Rezaei, F., Hosseini Ramaghani, N. A., & Fazio, R. L. (2017). The effect of a third party observer and trait anxiety on neuropsychological performance: The Attentional Control Theory (ACT) perspective. *The Clinical Neuropsychologist, 31*(3), 632–643. https://doi.org/10.1080/13854046.2016.1266031

Rodolfa, E., Hall, T., Holms, V., Davena, A., Komatz, D., Antunez, M., & Hall, A. (1994). The management of sexual feelings in therapy. *Professional Psychology: Research and Practice, 25*(2), 168–172. https://doi.org/10.1037/0735-7028.25.2.168

Rodriguez, N. (2014, July 2). Former U of L dean Robert Felner sentenced to 63 months in prison. *Courier Journal.* https://www.courier-journal.com/story/news/crime/2014/07/02/robert-felner-faces-63-months-in-prison-restitution/12064695/

Rogers, R., Tazi, K. Y., & Drogin, E. Y. (2023). Forensic assessment instruments: Their reliability and applicability to criminal forensic issues. *Behavioral Sciences & the Law, 41*(5), 415–431. https://doi.org/10.1002/bsl.2613

Ross, L. (1977). The intuitive psychologist and his shortcomings: Distortions in the attribution process. In L. Berkowitz (Ed.), *Advances in experimental social psychology* (Vol. 10, pp. 173–220). Academic Press. https://doi.org/10.1016/S0065-2601(08)60357-3

Ross, L. (2018). From the fundamental attribution error to the truly fundamental attribution error and beyond: My research journey. *Perspectives on Psychological Science, 13*(6), 750–769. https://doi.org/10.1177/1745691618769855

Roy v. Hartogs, 381 N. Y. S.2d 587 (1976).

Salmen, K., Ermark, F. K. G., & Fiedler, K. (2023). Pragmatic, constructive, and reconstructive memory influences on the hindsight bias. *Psychonomic Bulletin & Review, 30*(1), 331–340. https://doi.org/10.3758/s13423-022-02158-1

Sattar, S. P., Pinals, D. A., & Gutheil, T. (2002). Countering countertransference: A forensic trainee's dilemma. *Journal of the American Academy of Psychiatry and the Law, 30*(1), 65–69.

Schachter, A., Flores, R. D., & Maghbouleh, N. (2021). Ancestry, color, or culture? How Whites racially classify others in the U.S. *American Journal of Sociology, 126*(5), 1220–1263. https://doi.org/10.1086/714215

Schetky, D. H., & Colbach, E. M. (1982). Countertransference on the witness stand: A flight from self? *Bulletin of the American Academy of Psychiatry & the Law, 10*(2), 115–121.

Schoener, G. R., & Gonsiorek, J. (1988). Assessment and development of rehabilitation plans for counselors who have sexually exploited their clients. *Journal of Counseling & Development, 67*(4), 227–232. https://doi.org/10.1002/j.1556-6676.1988.tb02588.x

Scopelliti, I., Morewedge, C. K., McCormick, E., Min, H. L., Lebrecht, S., & Kassam, K. S. (2015). Bias blind spot: Structure, measurement, and consequences. *Management Science, 61*(10), 2468–2486. https://doi.org/10.1287/mnsc.2014.2096

Scurich, N., Güney, Ş., & Dietz, P. (2023). Hindsight bias in assessing child sexual abuse. *Journal of Sexual Aggression, 29*(1), 103–117. https://doi.org/10.1080/13552600.2022.2034999

Security and Privacy, 45 C.F.R. § 164.501 (2015).

Segal, S. J. (1971). *Imagery: Current cognitive approaches.* Academic Press.

Sehlmeyer v. Department of General Services, 17 Cal. App. 4 1072 (1993).

Sheehan, P. (1972). *The function and nature of imagery.* Academic Press.

Shepard, M. (1971). *The love treatment: Sexual intimacy between patients and psychotherapists.* Wyden.

Shepherd, M. (1975). *Fritz: An intimate portrait of Fritz Perls and Gestalt therapy.* Saturday Review Press.

Siegel, D. M., & Kinscherff, R. (2018). Recording routine forensic mental health evaluations should be a standard of practice in the 21st century. *Behavioral Sciences & the Law, 36*(3), 373–389. https://doi.org/10.1002/bsl.2349

Simon, R. I. (1999). Therapist–patient sex. From boundary violations to sexual misconduct. *Psychiatric Clinics of North America, 22*(1), 31–47. https://doi.org/10.1016/S0193-953X(05)70057-5

Singer, J. L. (1975a). *The inner world of daydreaming.* Harper & Row.

Singer, J. L. (1975b). Navigating the stream of consciousness: Research in daydreaming and related inner experiences. *American Psychologist, 30*(7), 727–738. https://doi.org/10.1037/h0076928

Singh, A., & dickey, l. m. (Eds.). (2017). *Affirmative counseling and psychological practice with transgender and gender nonconforming clients.* American Psychological Association. https://doi.org/10.1037/14957-000

Skinner, B. F. (1975). The steep and thorny way to a science of behavior. *American Psychologist, 30*(1), 42–49. https://doi.org/10.1037/0003-066X.30.1.42

Slochower, J. (2021). Don't tell anyone. In C. Levin (Ed.), *Sexual boundary trouble in psychoanalysis* (pp. 143–158). Taylor & Francis. Kindle Edition.

Slovic, P., & Fischhoff, B. (1977). On the psychology of experimental surprises. *Journal of Experimental Psychology: Human Perception and Performance, 3*(4), 544–551. https://doi.org/10.1037/0096-1523.3.4.544

Smedley, A., & Smedley, B. D. (2005). Race as biology is fiction, racism as a social problem is real: Anthropological and historical perspectives on the social construction of race. *American Psychologist, 60*(1), 16–26. https://doi.org/10.1037/0003-066X.60.1.16

Smith, S. (1989). The seduction of the female patient. In G. O. Gabbard (Ed.), *Sexual exploitation in professional relationships* (pp. 57–69). American Psychiatric Press.

Somer, E., & Saadon, M. (1999). Therapist-client sex: Clients' retrospective reports. *Professional Psychology: Research and Practice, 30*(5), 504–509. https://doi.org/10.1037/0735-7028.30.5.504

Sonne, J. L., & Jochai, D. (2014). The "vicissitudes of love" between therapist and patient: A review of the research on romantic and sexual feelings, thoughts, and behaviors in psychotherapy. *Journal of Clinical Psychology, 70*(2), 182–195. https://doi.org/10.1002/jclp.22069

Sonne, J., Meyer, C. B., Borys, D., & Marshall, V. (1985). Clients' reactions to sexual intimacy in therapy. *American Journal of Orthopsychiatry, 55*(2), 183–189. https://doi.org/10.1111/j.1939-0025.1985.tb03432.x

Stoute, B. J. (2020). Racism: A challenge for the therapeutic dyad. *American Journal of Psychotherapy, 73*(3), 69–71. https://doi.org/10.1176/appi.psychotherapy.20200043

Strasburger, L. H., Gutheil, T. G., & Brodsky, A. (1997). On wearing two hats: Role conflict in serving as both psychotherapist and expert witness. *The American Journal of Psychiatry, 154*(4), 448–456. https://doi.org/10.1176/ajp.154.4.448

Strean, H. S. (2018). *Therapists who have sex with their patients.* Routledge.

Sue, D. W., Rivera, D. P., Watkins, N. L., Kim, R. H., Kim, S., & Williams, C. D. (2011). Racial dialogues: Challenges faculty of color face in the classroom. *Cultural Diversity & Ethnic Minority Psychology, 17*(3), 331–340. https://doi.org/10.1037/a0024190

Sullivan, H. S. (1947). *Conceptions of modern psychiatry.* William Alanson White Psychiatric Foundation.

Taleb, N. N. (2010). *The black swan: The impact of the highly improbable fragility* (2nd ed.). Random House Trade Paperbacks.

Taleb, N. N., & Blyth, M. (2011, May/June). The black swan of Cairo: How suppressing volatility makes the world less predictable and more dangerous. *Foreign Affairs*, 33–39. https://www.foreignaffairs.com/articles/egypt/2011-06-01/black-swan-cairo

Tate, C. C., Youssef, C. P., & Bettergarcia, J. N. (2014). Integrating the study of transgender spectrum and cisgender experiences of self-categorization from a personality perspective. *Review of General Psychology, 18*(4), 302–312. https://doi.org/10.1037/gpr0000019

Tummala-Narra, P. (2021). Considering racial and cultural context in sexual boundary violations. In A. (L.) Steinberg, J. L. Alpert, & C. A. Courtois (Eds.), *Sexual boundary violations in psychotherapy: Facing therapist indiscretions, transgressions, and misconduct* (pp. 205–217). American Psychological Association. https://doi.org/10.1037/0000247-012

Unger, R. K. (1979). Toward a redefinition of sex and gender. *American Psychologist, 34*(11), 1085–1094. https://doi.org/10.1037/0003-066X.34.11.1085

U.S. Department of Health and Human Services. (2023). *Subpart E—Privacy of individually identifiable health information.* https://www.govinfo.gov/content/pkg/CFR-2023-title45-vol2/pdf/CFR-2023-title45-vol2-sec164-501.pdf

Utsey, S. O., Gernat, C. A., & Hammar, L. (2005). Examining White counselor trainees' reactions to racial issues in counseling and supervision dyads. *The Counseling Psychologist, 33*(4), 449–478. https://doi.org/10.1177/0011000004269058

Van Buren, A. (1978, June 11). "Dear Abby." *San Francisco Sunday Examiner and Chronicle,* p. 6.

Vesentini, L., Van Overmeire, R., Matthys, F., De Wachter, D., Van Puyenbroeck, H., & Bilsen, J. (2022). Intimacy in psychotherapy: An exploratory survey among therapists. *Archives of Sexual Behavior, 51*(1), 453–463. https://doi.org/10.1007/s10508-021-02190-7

Vesentini, L., Van Puyenbroeck, H., De Wachter, D., Matthys, F., & Bilsen, J. (2023). Managing romantic and sexual feelings towards clients in the psychotherapy room in Flanders (Belgium). *Sexual Abuse, 35*(3), 263–287. https://doi.org/10.1177/10790632221098357

Vinson, J. S. (1987). Use of complaint procedures in cases of therapist–patient sexual contact. *Professional Psychology: Research and Practice, 18*(2), 159–164. https://doi.org/10.1037/0735-7028.18.2.159

Waisman, J. C. (2017). *The intersection of professional boundaries and trauma in psychotherapy with adolescents: A preliminary study.* Smith College School for Social Work.

Walker, E., & Young, P. D. (1986). *A killing cure.* Holt.

Warner, S. L. (1994). Freud's analysis of Horace Frink, M.D.: A previously unexplained therapeutic disaster. *Psychodynamic Psychiatry, 22*(1), 137–152. https://doi.org/10.1521/jaap.1.1994.22.1.137

Watson, J. B. (1913). Psychology as the behaviorist views it. *Psychological Review, 20*(2), 158–177. https://doi.org/10.1037/h0074428

Watson, J. B. (1914). *Behavior: An introduction to comparative psychology.* Holt. https://doi.org/10.1037/10868-000

Watson, J. B. (1919). *Psychology from the standpoint of a behaviorist.* J. B. Lippincott. https://doi.org/10.1037/10016-000

Watson, J. B. (1925). *Behaviorism.* Norton.

Wellman, F. L. (1911). *The art of cross-examination* (new and enlarged ed.). The MacMillan Company.

Wenzlaff, F., Briken, P., & Dekker, A. (2018). If there's a penis, it's most likely a man: Investigating the social construction of gender using eye tracking. *PLOS ONE, 13*(3), Article e0193616. https://doi.org/10.1371/journal.pone.0193616

West, R. F., Meserve, R. J., & Stanovich, K. E. (2012). Cognitive sophistication does not attenuate the bias blind spot. *Journal of Personality and Social Psychology, 103*(3), 506–519. https://doi.org/10.1037/a0028857

Williams, D. J., & Sprott, R. A. (2022). Current biopsychosocial science on understanding kink. *Current Opinion in Psychology, 48*, Article 101473. https://doi.org/10.1016/j.copsyc.2022.101473

Wilson, G. D. (1997). Gender differences in sexual fantasy: An evolutionary analysis. *Personality and Individual Differences, 22*(1), 27–31. https://doi.org/10.1016/S0191-8869(96)00180-8

Wilson, G. D., & Lang, R. J. (1981). Sex differences in sexual fantasy patterns. *Personality and Individual Differences, 2*(4), 343–346. https://doi.org/10.1016/0191-8869(81)90093-3

Winnicott, D. W. (1965). *The maturational processes and the facilitating environment: Studies in the theory of emotional development.* International Universities Press.

Wood, G. (1978). The knew-it-all-along effect. *Journal of Experimental Psychology: Human Perception and Performance, 4*(2), 345–353. https://doi.org/10.1037/0096-1523.4.2.345

Yantz, C. L., & McCaffrey, R. J. (2009). Effects of parental presence and child characteristics on children's neuropsychological test performance: Third party observer effect confirmed. *The Clinical Neuropsychologist, 23*(1), 118–132. https://doi.org/10.1080/13854040801894722

Yi, J., Neville, H. A., Todd, N. R., & Mekawi, Y. (2023). Ignoring race and denying racism: A meta-analysis of the associations between colorblind racial ideology, anti-Blackness, and other variables antithetical to racial justice. *Journal of Counseling Psychology, 70*(3), 258–275. https://doi.org/10.1037/cou0000618

Yule, M. A., Brotto, L. A., & Gorzalka, B. B. (2017). Sexual fantasy and masturbation among asexual individuals: An in-depth exploration. *Archives of Sexual Behavior, 46*(1), 311–328. https://doi.org/10.1007/s10508-016-0870-8

Zaleskiewicz, T., & Gasiorowska, A. (2021). Evaluating experts may serve psychological needs: Self-esteem, bias blind spot, and processing fluency explain confirmation effect in assessing financial advisors' authority. *Journal of Experimental Psychology: Applied, 27*(1), 27–45. https://doi.org/10.1037/xap0000308

Zapf, P. A., Kukucka, J., Kassin, S. M., & Dror, I. E. (2018). Cognitive bias in forensic mental health assessment: Evaluator beliefs about its nature and scope. *Psychology, Public Policy, and Law, 24*(1), 1–10. https://doi.org/10.1037/law0000153

Zipkin v. Freeman, 436 S. W. 2d 753 (Mo. 1968).

Zwartz, M. (2018). Report writing in the forensic context: Recurring problems and the use of a checklist to address them. *Psychiatry, Psychology and Law, 25*(4), 578–588. https://doi.org/10.1080/13218719.2018.1473172

Index

and information collected during
assessment, 93, 95
informed consent on limitations of,
95, 121
legally recognized exceptions to, 152n3
motion to quash citing, 149
negotiations with requester of
information over, 148
opposing release of information on
grounds of, 151–152
Therapist–patient sexual involvement, 9
colleague betrayal with, 56–57
coming to terms with psychology's
history of, 21–22
contemporary views of sex and gender
in, 40–41
contemporary views of sexuality in,
41–45
emotional reactions to allegations of,
104–106
expert testimony on, 85
gender of patients who engage in, 37–38
gender of therapists who engage in,
36–37
harm caused by. *See* Patient harm from
therapist–patient sex
impact of, on others in therapist's life,
56–57
influential therapists who engaged in,
3–4, 16–22, 103–104
lawsuits over, 22, 23, 99, 122.
See also Forensic work involving
therapist–patient sex
media portrayals of, 22, 23
other psychologist's reactions to, 20–21
prohibitions on, 16
race in, 45–47
raising awareness of, 22–23
research on, 8, 51–53
results of, for therapist, 59
self-reflections on, 11–12, 24
subsequent clinical work with patients
who experience. *See* Clinical
work with patients with history of
therapist–patient sex
testifying about. *See* Forensic testimony
therapist vulnerabilities for. *See* Therapist
vulnerabilities for therapist–patient sex
Therapist's role
conflict related to, 88–89, 120
as source of power, 34

Therapist vulnerabilities for therapist–
patient sex, 21, 59–68
awareness of, 64
character disorders with impulse
control, 65–66
with child and adolescent patients, 66
gender, 66–67
grandiosity and self-centeredness,
64–65
isolation, 62–63
loneliness, 60–62
neediness, 63–64
powerful, persistent, or indulged
fantasies about client, 60
self-reflection on, 67–68
Third parties
confidentiality issues for, 147
informed consent and, 95, 120
protective order for, 149
threats to, 93
"Third Party Observers" (Gavett et al.),
95
Third-party payment sources, 120, 129
Transference, 17
Transgender people, 36, 40
"Trauma-Informed Forensic Mental
Health Assessment: Practical
Implications, Ethical Tensions,
and Alignment with Therapeutic
Jurisprudence Standards"
(Goldenson et al.), 79
Treatment plan, 125–126, 128
Trust, 21, 33–34
Truth, 72

U

Undocumented migrants, 12–13
Undue burden or expense, with subpoena,
153, 162
Unmet needs, 31, 60–61, 63–64
Unusual sexual fantasies, 26
Use of Assessment (Standard 9.02), 159
"Using the MMPI-3 in Legal Settings"
(Ben-Porath et al.), 78

V

Validity, assessment instrument, 94
Vasquez, M. J. T., 86–87
Vesentini, L., 28, 29

Victim blaming, 55, 109
Videoconferencing, 95
Vienna Psychoanalytic Society, 17

W

Walker, E., 22
Watson, John B., 17
Watterson, K., 22
Wellman, F. L., 102–103
We–they attitude, 56
What you see is all there is (WYSIATI),
    16, 110
Williams, D. J., 26
Winnicott, D. W., 64
Women of Color, 36, 46. *See also* Female-
    identifying people and women

WYSIATI (what you see is all there is),
    16, 110

Y

You Must Be Dreaming (Noël & Watterson),
    22–23
Young, P. D., 22

Z

Zapf, P. A., 102
Zelen, S. L., 63
Zipkin v. Freeman, 22
Zoom, 9, 95
Zwartz, M., 96

About the Authors

Kenneth S. Pope, PhD, ABPP, is a licensed psychologist. A fellow of the Association for Psychological Science, he served as chair of the ethics committees of the American Board of Professional Psychology (ABPP) and the American Psychological Association (APA). He received the APA Award for Distinguished Contributions to Public Service, the APA Division 12 (Society of Clinical Psychology) Award for Distinguished Professional Contributions to Clinical Psychology, the Canadian Psychological Association's John C. Service Member of the Year Award, and the Ontario Psychological Association's Barbara Wand Award for significant contribution to excellence in professional ethics and standards. Dr. Pope's authored or coauthored books include *Speaking the Unspoken: Breaking the Silence, Myths, and Taboos That Hurt Therapists and Patients* (with Nayeli Y. Chavez-Dueñas, Hector Y. Adames, Janet L. Sonne, and Beverly A. Greene, 2023); *Succeeding as a Therapist: How to Create a Thriving Practice in a Changing World* (with Hector Y. Adames, Nayeli Y. Chavez-Dueñas, and Melba J. T. Vasquez, 2023); the sixth edition of *Ethics in Psychotherapy and Counseling: A Practical Guide* (with Melba J. T. Vasquez, Nayeli Y. Chavez-Dueñas, and Hector Y. Adames, 2021); *Five Steps to Strengthen Ethics in Organizations and Individuals: Effective Strategies Informed by Research and History* (2017); the third edition of *The MMPI, MMPI-2, and MMPI-A in Court: A Practical Guide for Expert Witnesses and Attorneys* (with James N. Butcher and Joyce Seelen, 2006); *What Therapists Don't Talk About and Why: Understanding Taboos That Hurt Us and Our Clients* (with Janet L. Sonne and Beverly Greene, 2006); *How to Survive and Thrive as a Therapist: Information, Ideas, and Resources for Psychologists in Practice* (with Melba J. T. Vasquez, 2005); *Recovered Memories of Abuse: Assessment, Therapy, Forensics* (with Laura S. Brown, 1996); *Sexual Involvement With Therapists: Patient Assessment, Subsequent Therapy, Forensics* (1994); *Sexual Feelings in*

Psychotherapy: Explorations for Therapists and Therapists-in-Training (with Janet L. Sonne and Jean Holroyd, 1993); and *Sexual Intimacy Between Therapists and Patients* (with Jacqueline C. Bouhoutsos, 1986).

Nayeli Y. Chavez-Dueñas, PhD, received her doctorate in clinical psychology from the American Psychological Association (APA)-accredited program at Southern Illinois University Carbondale. She is a professor at The Chicago School, College of Professional Psychology, where she is the lead for the concentration in Latinx mental health in the Counseling Psychology Department. She also is the cofounder and codirector of the IC-RACE Lab (Immigration Critical Race and Cultural Equity Lab). Dr. Chavez-Dueñas has coauthored several books: *Speaking the Unspoken: Breaking the Silence, Myths, and Taboos That Hurt Therapists and Patients* (with Kenneth S. Pope, Hector Y. Adames, Janet L. Sonne, and Beverly A. Greene, 2023); *Succeeding as a Therapist: How to Create a Thriving Practice in a Changing World* (with Hector Y. Adames, Melba J. T. Vasquez, and Kenneth S. Pope, 2023); the sixth edition of *Ethics in Psychotherapy and Counseling: A Practical Guide* (with Kenneth S. Pope, Melba J. T. Vasquez, and Hector Y. Adames, 2021); and *Cultural Foundations and Interventions in Latino/a Mental Health: History, Theory, and Within-Group Differences* (with Hector Y. Adames, 2017). She recently coedited the book *Decolonial Psychology: Toward Anticolonial Theories, Research, Training, and Practice* (with Lillian Comas-Díaz and Hector Y. Adames, 2024). Her research focuses on colorism, skin-color differences, parenting styles, immigration, unaccompanied minors, multiculturalism, and race relations. She has earned a number of awards, including the 2018 APA Distinguished Citizen Psychologist Award and the 2023 Distinguished Professional Career Award from the National Latinx Psychological Association. Visit https://icrace.org/ for more information about her lab.

Hector Y. Adames, PsyD, received his doctorate in clinical psychology from the American Psychological Association (APA)-accredited program at Wright State University in Ohio and completed his APA predoctoral internship at the Boston University School of Medicine Center for Multicultural Training in Psychology. Currently, he is a licensed psychologist and a professor at The Chicago School, College of Professional Psychology, and the cofounder and codirector of the IC-RACE Lab (Immigration Critical Race and Cultural Equity Lab). Dr. Adames has coauthored several books, including *Speaking the Unspoken: Breaking the Silence, Myths, and Taboos That Hurt Therapists and Patients* (with Kenneth S. Pope, Nayeli Y. Chavez-Dueñas, Janet L. Sonne, and Beverly A. Greene, 2023); *Succeeding as a*

Therapist: How to Create a Thriving Practice in a Changing World (with Nayeli Y. Chavez-Dueñas, Melba J. T. Vasquez, and Kenneth S. Pope, 2023); the sixth edition of *Ethics in Psychotherapy and Counseling: A Practical Guide* (with Kenneth S. Pope, Melba J. T. Vasquez, and Nayeli Y. Chavez-Dueñas, 2021); and *Cultural Foundations and Interventions in Latino/a Mental Health: History, Theory, and Within-Group Differences* (with Nayeli Y. Chavez-Dueñas, 2017). He has also coedited two books, *Decolonial Psychology: Toward Anticolonial Theories, Research, Training, and Practice* (with Lillian Comas-Díaz and Nayeli Y. Chavez-Dueñas, 2024) and *Caring for Latinxs With Dementia in a Globalized World: Behavioral and Psychosocial Treatments* (with Yvette N. Tazeau, 2020). He has earned several awards, including the 2018 Distinguished Emerging Professional Research Award from the Society for the Psychological Study of Culture, Ethnicity, and Race (APA Division 45) and a 2021 Presidential Citation award by APA. Visit https://icrace.org/ to learn more about his lab.